LAST WISH

Stories to Inspire
a Peaceful Passing

Lauren Van Scoy, M.D.

TRANSMEDIA BOOKS and colophon are trademarks
of Amicus Partners, Inc.
For information regarding special discounts for bulk purchases,
please contact Transmedia Books Special Sales at
1-858-756-5767 or sales@TransmediaBooks.com.
TRANSMEDIA BOOKS
3525 Del Mar Heights Rd. Suite 111
San Diego, CA 92130-2122

Cover Designed by Pitkow Associates
Manufactured in the United States of America
Library of Congress Control Number 2012936954

ISBN-13: 978-0-9834511-9-8
ISBN-10: 0983451192

Discussion Questions Developed and Written by Alicia Bloom

Alicia Marini Bloom, MSW LSW is a masters-prepared, licensed social worker that has been practicing in hospice & palliative care for over six years in both the inpatient & outpatient settings. Currently, she works for VITAS Innovative Hospice Care—the nation's leading hospice provider. In her role, Alicia has the privilege of providing direct care to patients and their families, and focuses on clinical education of healthcare providers and the community at large about hospice and palliative care to increase access and utilization of critically important services to people living with serious illness and their families. A graduate of the University of Pennsylvania with a BA in Sociology and a Masters of Social Work, Alicia is published in the International Journal of Palliative Nursing for her experience as part of a clinical team that developed and implemented a palliative care educational program at the University of Botswana. She is also published in the Journal of Palliative Medicine.

Praise For Last Wish: Stories To Inspire A Peaceful Passing

"...a must read for all thoughtful adults"

"*Last Wish* is a must-read for all thoughtful adults. The book reads like a bestseller, but its honesty about the final decision of a lifetime is a mosaic of emotion that shocks you, enlightens you, and in poignant and memorable true stories, Ultimately sets you free."

~ **Larry Kane, Anchor, Author, and TV Host**

"...sheds new light on an old, and often avoided conversation"

"We will all face end of life decisions, but most don't give the matters thought until we are in crisis. Better to face the tough decisions when we are of sound body and mind than to await our eventual fate. By offering vignettes and compelling facts, Dr. Van Scoy sheds new light on an old, and often avoided conversation."

~ **Michael A. Smerconish, nationally syndicated radio talk show host**

"...highly recommended for all who will likely face these choices for a loved one, and inevitably someday for ourselves."

"To be a professional advocate for research for healthier and more vital aging does not mean one favors life extension at any cost. I read Dr. Van Scoy's engrossing book on a cross-country flight to visit my 94-year-old mother, quite possibly for the last time. Therefore, the end-of-life issues that are so wisely and humanly considered in Last Wish were very much on my mind.

"I find myself in deep sympathy and respect for the patients, families and health professionals who are vividly portrayed in these vignettes. Alas, the pursuit of the "good death" remains as elusive as ever, and is made even more difficult by the painful dilemmas often thrust upon us by modern intensive care technology.

"The stories told in these pages, together with the resources and web-based supports offered at the end, are highly recommended for all who will likely face these choices for a loved one, and inevitably someday for ourselves."

"The stories told in these pages, together with the resources and web-based supports offered at the end, are highly recommended for all who will likely face these choices for a loved one, and inevitably someday for ourselves."

~ Daniel Perry, President and CEO, Alliance for Aging Research

"...the stories are as entertaining a read as they are thought-provoking."

"Dr. Van Scoy's collection of real-life case scenarios of patients and their families who were faced with these decisions provides insights and perspectives that are useful to laymen and healthcare providers alike. The value of the patients' stories is enhanced by the first-hand insights provided from the perspective of a young house officer providing care to these critically ill patients with a heart of passion, but the naïveté that permits a close connection with the difficult predicament the families are facing. Always serious and passionate, the stories are as entertaining a read as they are thought-provoking. It is an outstanding read and a valuable asset to this literature."

~ James C. Reynolds, M.D., June F. Klinghoffer, Distinguished Professor and Chair, Dept. of Medicine, Drexel University College of Medicine

"...highly recommended for all who will likely face these choices for a loved one, and inevitably someday for ourselves."

"This is an important book that tells the stories of how people choose to die and how their families are affected. It discusses the importance of knowing when to pursue aggressive therapies and when it is reasonable to stop and allow natural death. It should be read by people with chronic illness making tough choices on their own end-of-life decisions. It should be read by family members of hospitalized patients in intensive care units. It should be read by policymakers and politicians. It should be read by all of us, who will someday be confronting our own mortality."

Michael Sherman, M.D., Author of The Pocket Doctor (Informa Healthcare 2002), Associate Professor of Medicine and Program Director, Pulmonary and Critical Care Fellowship, Drexel University College of Medicine

"Beautifully, thoughtfully and respectfully written..."

"Emily Dickinson wrote, 'Unable are the loved to die/For love is immortality...' In her book 'Last Wish' Van Scoy shows us the truth of this statement. In a vivid narrative the author guides us through stories of five people and their loved ones facing death. These stories don't just paint a realistic picture of the complexity of end-of-life decisions and discussions for families. They also show with honesty and respect the rock-tumbler of medical training, where every-day intensity can either smooth out the rough edges or grind you to dust. Dr. Van Scoy's book took me back to my training in ICU medicine, and reminded me that the lines of separation we draw ~ you patient, me doctor ~ are arbitrary, and that we are all bound by our humanity, so palpably present at the time of dying."

~ Marya Zilberberg, MD, MPH, FCCP, Founder, President and CEO, EviMed Research Group, LLC; Associate Professor of Epidemiology, School of Public Health and Health Sciences, University of Massachusetts, Amherst; author of "Between the Lines: Finding the Truth in Medical Literature

"a book that boils all the Hollywood out of ER, House, Scrubs... leaving the raw reality of the difficult times that come at the end of human life.

~ Andrew Hill, staff writer, Geekadelphia website

"So compellingly written is DNR that – once begun –I had to read it straight through..."

~ Kathy Kastner, Publisher and Editor, Ability4Life.org

"...the stories are told with grace, respect and empathy. They made me more aware of the complex issues involved in end of life care and decisions.

To the memory of
Dianne Ball

Contents

Foreword

A few years ago, my friend Mathew Holt and I met for dinner, the kind of dinner where food is the side and the main course is a fully engrossing conversation that barrels along a mile a minute. We wound our way onto the topic of end of life care and jointly bemoaned how terribly our country deals with it. We considered the statistics, like the fact that 70 percent of people want to die at home but only 30 percent do. And then, because life is about a lot more than statistics, we started sharing our stories. And when it was my turn, I decided to share the story of my sister-in-law, Za.

The week before my wedding, my fiancé's sister Za, whom I had come to feel was my sister, fell ill. Not regular, run-of-the-mill ill, but *ill* ill. She was tired and despondent, even surly, sometimes. Their two-year-old daughter, Alessia, was confused.

On the day Antonio and I were to be married, the entire family, some fresh off the plane from Sicily, read Za the riot act. "Come on. You need to pull up your socks and get it together. Tonight is a big event, and you need to be there." We sent her off to the local hospital to be hydrated, since clearly this was just an issue of Za not taking care of herself, nothing a few liters of IV fluid wouldn't fix. She was a dedicated pharmacist who worked many hours at her job, and the mother of a two-year-old daughter besides. Who wouldn't be run down?

While we were busying ourselves with final preparations, a concerned care team took Za in for an MRI.

While we were heading to our ceremony, the doctors conferred over a mass in her brain.

As our reception was beginning, we were toasting how much we missed Za, and how sad we were that she seemed to have some bad flu or perhaps even mono. Meanwhile, she was rushed by ambulance to Massachusetts General Hospital.

The next morning, we received the call. Za was in a coma-like state, unable to communicate, speaking only in Italian, which neither the nurses nor her husband, John, understood. Within a nanosecond, we checked out of our romantic, wedding-night hotel and checked in to what was to become our reality for the next seven months.

When we got to the hospital, my new husband went immediately to Za's side, working to understand what no one could comprehend: *la testa, ma testa . . . dolore dolore.* She was repeating it over and over: "the head, my head . . . the pain, the pain."

I'll never forget how the surgeon looked when I approached him outside her room to ask him what was happening to Za, the way the light hit his face, the way the shadow on the computer screen *almost* masked what I didn't want to see. Yet what I remember most is the kindness in his eyes, the humanity as he told me, "What you are looking at is glioblastoma, and I think it's stage four."

Months passed before we as a family actually discussed, out loud, what I feared to even think of that day as I stood talking to the surgeon. Za didn't have long to live. She was 32.

During this time, our family cultivated a balance of responsibility. My job was to question authority, and Antonio's was to ignore it. While Antonio was the emotional link that helped Za communicate with the rest of us, I took on the role that my job running a young healthcare company had trained me for: not taking anything for granted, even in a hospital environment. I spent hours conferring with the doctors, consulting my network of industry gurus, constantly running statistics through my head.

By June, following two surgeries, radiation, and chemotherapy, Za's cancer had spread to her back. We knew what this meant for her. She didn't have long left. But what did this mean for her daughter, Alessia, who was only two years old? Well, in the beginning it meant something wonderful: Mama quit work! Yet over time, it began to mean that Mama didn't feel well, Mama couldn't walk, and Mama couldn't speak.

Za spent the last two months of her life in a hospital bed, and while we were with her every night to regale her with tales of our day, Alessia withdrew. After all, what do tubes and shaved heads and funny smells mean when you are two years old? Nothing good, that's for sure.

When the end was near, the doctors pulled us aside and advised us of the options. They strongly suggested we keep her in the hospital to make sure she would be well cared for. They worried that her case was so complex that there was no way we could care for her at home.

Instead of pushing back, I suddenly became the acceptor of our fate, convincing myself and my family that Za should stay in the hospital. I, the one who until this point had always questioned, always pushed, was now resigned. And so our roles changed. Antonio, who had been raised not to question the word of a doctor suddenly became a completely different person.

When we met with her oncologists to decide Za's fate, most of us believed the doctors when they told us bringing Za home would be an incredible mistake. But Antonio's response?

"Of course, and unquestionably, we are taking her home," he said.

So we did.

And that night, after two months in the hospital, two long months of Alessia feeling afraid to hug, lie next to, talk to or touch this mum she had stopped being able to recognize—on the very first night we had Za settled at home, safely surrounded by the comforts, the familiarities and smells of those four sacred walls—Alessia, for the first time in eight weeks, crawled up next to her in the bed and gave her mum her medicine. And Za, who had not spoken or opened her eyes in at least a week, woke up fully, looked her daughter square in the eyes, and loved her in the way that only a mum can. The next night Za died, peacefully, at home.

I sometimes wonder who received the greatest gift that night. Was it Za, who may finally have felt some peace, at home, finally able to connect with her daughter? Or was it Alessia, who is now eight and still to this day crawls into my lap to hear stories of her mum and how she was the very last thing her mum held that night? Or was it really the rest of us, honored to witness that incredible moment, knowing now we almost missed it?

And so, as our food got cold, Matthew and I dreamed up a movement which became Engage with Grace, our mission being to make people think about these tough questions before it's too late.

Our approach is simple, a bid to get folks to answer just five questions that would be useful to know should they ever suffer an advanced illness or end-of-life situation. Simplicity is the point, our concern being that the complexity of many of the advance directives and documents that exist today overwhelm those who attempt to document their preferences and choices. Engage with Grace was designed to make sure everyone has the gift of a life lived fully and in the way they intend.

We set out to ask just five simple questions, which can be found in the Resources section in the back of this book. Our goal is to get folks talking about topics we naturally tend to avoid thinking about, like "What if I, or someone I love fiercely, gets really sick, and it's up to me to make decisions for them? What would I do and, more important, what would *they* want me to do?" Alternatively, if you ever found yourself in this place to which few of us aspire, would you be cared for in the way that you hope, in a way that aligns with your values and wishes?

Reading this book by Dr. Van Scoy, (or LJ to those of us who know her), it struck me: while simplicity can help to get that incredibly important conversation started, life and serious illness *isn't* always so simple. And this is where *Last Wish* becomes an invaluable resource for all of us facing our inevitable mortality. This book gives us the insight we need to confront the five questions of Engage With Grace, remembering that there are no wrong answers. It's only wrong if no one *knows* your answer and cannot advocate for you. Since we launched Engage With Grace, we've found that once the conversation starts and our thoughts and wishes are shared with those we love, then the system that intervenes to bowl over our intent stops being intimidating and we become empowered.

Once you start reading *Last Wish*, I promise, you will not be able to stop. As you read, you'll make mental notes to be sure you never do this or always do that. And if someone tries to interrupt you while you're in the middle of one of the stories, you'll feel a tiny bit of annoyance that you'll try to hide. You'll find that you've emerged on the other side wiser, more nuanced and sensitive to just how *not* simple all aspects of life, including this one, can be. And that awareness just might give you the clarity of purpose to make sure your story ends the way you want it to.

ALEXANDRA DRANE

Introduction

As a doctor reaching the end of a 24-hour shift in the intensive care unit it's usually easy to fall asleep. The exhaustion hits you like a rock and it doesn't matter that the morning sun is pouring into your bedroom. After 24 long hours of fighting for life and pushing back against death, you finally hit your bed, close your eyes and, in an instant, the next day has arrived. Except for that one day when I couldn't sleep no matter what I tried. Saddened from seeing the same turmoil time and time again as my patients' family members were caught unprepared, confused and distraught amidst an unexpected medical disaster, I tossed and turned in bed with an idea. I would write the stories of my patients so others might learn from their victories, struggles and even their failures. That night, I determined to write *Last Wish* to encourage you to consider in advance what your wishes, or those of your loved ones, might be if faced with an unexpected tragedy. I didn't sleep at all that day, despite my overwhelming fatigue, because the stories in my head kept me awake, begging to be written.

In the intensive care unit, I find myself talking with people every day about devastating illness, the fragility of our bodies, and our mortality. Options are presented: should we pursue aggressive, possibly painful interventions or perhaps shift our focus and allow a natural and peaceful passing? Without exception, it's agonizing for families to discuss a loved one's care in terms of pros and cons, possible outcomes, and life expectancy measured in months or less. There are lots of questions, and at the end, it usually comes down to them asking me just one more: "What should we do?"

It's an impossible question, and I have to give an impossible answer. *It's up to you.* As a doctor, all I can offer are choices and guidance, not a decision.

In the ICU, we're faced with the sickest patients, those with chronic and incurable diseases that have begun to advance and rage beyond control. We resuscitate and stabilize, dodging bullets and saving lives for the moment as patients and their families try to adjust to the trauma of it all, only to be left with another conundrum: now what?

So I wrote *Last Wish* intending to plant a seed in your mind about some of the medical situations you or your loved ones probably will face one day. Maybe it will provide some insight for you and your family. At the very least, I hope it sparks discussion and helps you to consider planning for the inevitable mortality we all face.

Yet *Last Wish* isn't about advance directives or other official documents and instructions. It's not even really about death, but instead about the incredible stories of five people who, through their courage, conviction, and spirit, can serve as inspiration for those who are either thinking ahead or struggling with approaching mortality right now.

Here, just as with my patients, I'm not advocating for any particular decision, but instead that you consider the issues. The decisions are yours and yours alone. No one can make them for you.

In this book, you'll read other people's experiences along with my own struggles with how to best treat the patient and support the family, and not always getting it right the first time. It's all told through my eyes and filled out with what I've learned from talking with the people involved. Indeed, it's my pleasure to introduce you to Bruce, Mrs. Chandler, Walter, Patrick and Victoria, all of whom are real people with important stories to share: stories of life, death and somewhere in-between.

1

A Biker's Heart

Bruce was a self-proclaimed rebel. In his youth, he found himself in and out of trouble since he walked a delicate line where the law was concerned. His greatest pleasure was his motorcycle. He'd gotten his first motorized bike, a moped, at age fifteen, and on it went from there as he'd trade up to bigger and bigger bikes until he owned the largest one he could get. Harleys, although he loved them, were just too small for Bruce. So he chose a bike that was not only bigger but also louder and stronger, and the roar of the engine matched his massive body and his muscular build. You could hear him coming from far away, and the ladies clapped their hands over their ears as he'd ride through town and flash a defiant smile of satisfaction.

Bruce's parents weren't as irked by his motorcycles as his neighbors were, but Bruce knew he wasn't a golden child. He left that role to his brother, Joseph, the son his mother had always wanted. Joseph had been college-bound and deeply religious in a way Bruce never was. Whereas Bruce always resisted going to church, Joseph had gone willingly and even spoken of studying religion once he was accepted to college. Well aware of the stark contrast between himself and Joseph, Bruce had also known that his parents always accepted him for who he was. College simply hadn't made his list of priorities. Unlike Joseph, Bruce hadn't planned out the rest of his life, but he'd landed a steady job at a local printing company and was known as a responsible and reliable worker. Right after high school, the extent of his long-range goals had been to work hard and ride his bike into the future.

He met Sharon while they were both working the night shift at the press when she was seventeen and he was twenty-one. The boss introduced them on her first day there, and after just one look, Bruce stuck out his hand and said, "Glad to meet you. Will you go out with me?"

Sharon was taken aback. She put him off, as she had to do some investigation about this Bruce character, but eventually, she agreed to go out on a date with him after her co-workers gave him the thumbs up. Three weeks later, he walked her to her car after a late shift and asked her to marry him. She said yes without hesitation, and their wedding soon thereafter surely raised some eyebrows in their small town in Pennsylvania.

Forty years and four kids later, I would meet Sharon in Bruce's room in the cardiac care unit, since she had never left his side since.

When I met him, Bruce's bravado had evaporated, and his vulnerability was overwhelming. With his abdomen exposed, a sterile dressing and my gloves were all that lay between my hands and his organs. Pressing carefully, I watched his face closely for a grimace that would indicate any pain breaking through his sedation. As his on-call doctor in the Cardiac Care Unit that night, I not only wanted to evaluate his discomfort to make sure we had the sedation just right. The goal was to keep the level not so high so that he was in a deep medically induced coma, and not so little so that he would become anxious and fight the ventilator as the machine did his breathing for him. It was a delicate balance.

Before they'd gone home, Bruce's daytime physicians had explained to me that his heart was failing and that he had a large sternal wound from his last open-heart surgery. He now had an infection, but not just any infection—it was The Infection, a murderously resistant one that was just as likely to kill him as it was to respond to antibiotics.

To enter his room, I'd had to follow isolation precautions lest I transfer his super-organism to another patient. I'd washed my hands, put on a yellow isolation gown and gloves, and then gone in to get my lay of the land. All the alarms and beeps were as they should be. The drips whirred softly on their pumps as they medicated Bruce to keep him alive. He had five bags of medication in all: two to keep his blood pressure from bottoming out, one for IV fluid, and two with the strongest antibiotics we had in our arsenal.

As an intern just out of medical school, I was on a four-week rotation in this unit. My seniors were just a phone call away, but somehow that wasn't very reassuring. Bruce was hanging between life and death, and if he started to swing in the wrong direction, it would be my job to notice and alert my senior resident. Yet if things went downhill, there wasn't much more we could do *besides* notice. So, covered head to toe in my yellow get-up, I stood checking things out, observing Bruce's baseline. *Some baseline*, I thought. His blood pressure teetered between "low" and "very low." His fever was a mere 101, and the ventilator was at its maximum settings.

Sadly, I didn't think Bruce would ever open his eyes again, and I didn't bother speaking to him since he probably couldn't hear me anyway, not through the drug-induced coma. Because his infection was too dangerous for me to risk contaminating my own stethoscope, I opened the packaging on a brand new plastic one and placed it on his chest, then listened for a heartbeat. So far, so good. His lungs sounded crackly, but the ventilator curves on the computer printout looked textbook perfect. Checking the surgical vacuum sucking the infection from his belly, my eyes followed the length of the tube connecting it to the container beside his bed and checked to make sure it hadn't suddenly filled with blood. Again, so far, so good. There was about a half cup of ooze, the same as in the morning.

The TV on Bruce's wall was tuned to the local news, and Bruce and I watched TV "together" for a few seconds. The top story was about yet another murder in West Philly, and I sighed, tired of the same headlines every night. Taking the remote from the bedside table, I switched it to the hospital music channel, dropped my gown into the hazardous waste bin, and went on to visit my next patient.

Bruce didn't die that night. Or the next. Instead, he stayed in that same tenuous state the entire time I was in my CCU rotation, and for a while afterward. While I was there, you could pretty much find Bruce lingering between life and death at any given moment but, other than that small but crucial detail, he was "stable." Months later, if you'd asked me, I would have told you I was sure that Bruce was dead.

At age 48, Bruce's first heart attack had led to his first open heart surgery. The first time his chest was cut open, a bypass operation restored blood flow to his heart, and the docs put in a defibrillator, a device that sat under his skin on his chest wall and would deliver a shock to his heart if it went into a deadly arrhythmia. He dealt with all of it well, and his recovery was rather uneventful. Just weeks later, he was back on his motorcycle, which he would ride to his monthly visits to his doctors.

It wasn't until Thanksgiving that things began to change. Bruce was sitting on the sofa and watching television, flanked by family members and his massive dogs. He felt a tickle in his hand where he held the remote. He dropped it onto the sofa, thinking it was giving some kind of electrical feedback as he was trying to turn up the volume on the football game. His wife and kids giggled at how a little static electricity got Big Bruce in such a tizzy. But it wasn't the remote; it was his defibrillator, and they figured that out just as soon as the second shock rendered him unconscious.

Two weeks later, Bruce was lying in his hospital bed listening to Dr. Farber rattle off a bunch of words that didn't make a whole lot of sense. *Transplant list. LVAD. Bridge therapy.* Sharon, as always, was by his side, looking equally dazed. They had gotten used to the term *CHF*, which stands for congestive heart failure. They had gotten used to *heart disease*. The word *transplant* just didn't seem relevant, though. Bruce didn't think he was that sick. He knew his heart was not in great condition, but a transplant? Impossible. Then, as with everything tough in his life, Bruce shrugged it off and plugged away. He'd get on the list. He'd get a new heart. It would be no big deal. His denial would get him through it all, and Sharon was right there with him. That was all he really needed anyway.

Dr. Farber's office ran like a well-oiled machine. She was one of the most highly celebrated heart failure doctors in the region, and her office routinely prepared patients for the LVAD surgery. They had case managers, nurse practitioners, cardiology fellows, and medical residents. They had surgeons and psychiatrists, all ready to guide Bruce and his family through the process. But first, there was a lot to explain.

LVAD stands for left ventricular assist device, something used in the direst of circumstances. It's a mechanical pump implanted directly into the heart to boost its pumping action, but it's certainly no artificial heart or miracle. It's a machine the patient becomes entirely dependent upon, requiring an external device to be worn at all times. Tubes running from the external device to the internal LVAD opens avenues for infection, blood clots, bleeding, and countless other deadly complications. The device is so complicated that they don't even teach you about it in medical school, as it's too daunting for medical students to truly grasp how it works. Dr. Farber's office staff had to explain it to Bruce, and all their other patients, and make certain that they understood exactly what they were about to embark upon.

For some patients, the LVAD is a bridge to transplant, a temporary measure to sustain their life until a donor heart becomes available. For others, it is a destination, the end of the road, the last chance for survival. For those patients who aren't candidates for a heart transplant, it's the only alternative to death.

Dr. Farber reviewed Bruce's hospital chart, muttering to herself as she flipped through the pages. She scanned his numbers and thought that Bruce would be a tough case. First, he had to overcome his lifestyle: he was overweight and a poorly controlled diabetic, a terrible combination for a transplant candidate. Second, she knew he was going to be waiting for a heart for a long, long time. Bruce's body habitus wasn't what one would call typical—rather, he was a big guy, and a donor heart had to be the correct size. Bruce would have to wait for an *extra*-large person of the right compatibility to die, and for that person to be an organ donor. Still, Dr. Farber had been around the transplant block and seen stranger things happen. She reviewed his prior echocardiograms and catheterizations and decided how best to medically manage Bruce while he waited for his precious donor heart.

Dr. Farber knew she had a job ahead of her in getting Bruce ready for the LVAD. She had to get him stable enough that his sick heart could endure the open-heart surgery required to place the LVAD so he had a chance of making it until a heart became available—if one became available. During her rounds, she checked on Bruce every day and tweaked his medical regimen just as frequently, based on the severity of his symptoms and the abnormalities on his labs. The transplant nutritionist counselled Bruce over and over about reducing his blood sugar and avoiding carbohydrate-rich foods, but it took a while to get Bruce to understand that his whole life needed to change. He was stubborn, rebellious, and incredibly tough. Dr. Farber knew he could do it; he just needed time to adjust. And he needed a good kick in the butt from his wife. Sharon, Dr. Farber knew, would do just that.

After a few weeks in the hospital, it was time. Dr. Farber couldn't wait any longer. Bruce's symptoms were getting progressively worse and he was struggling to breathe. They had to put in the LVAD.

While in the hospital, Bruce met several other patients in his unit with diseases and situations similar to his own. Scott, another heart failure patient, had received his LVAD a year ago. Bruce met Scott in the CCU and was shocked at how sick he was. Talking with Scott and his family helped Bruce to understand what to expect with this new addition to his life. Scott told him all about the surgery, the recovery, and how the LVAD had affected him: it was an incredible nuisance and had uprooted Scott's life to the fullest extent, but it had given him a chance to get on the transplant list and to survive. *Survive.* That was all Bruce needed to hear.

It was the second time they would crack open his chest, but he wasn't about to give in to his heart disease, and he knew there wasn't much choice in the matter. Maybe his course would be easier than poor Scott's. So Bruce got his LVAD without any problems, and his cardiac rehabilitation began.

Although the surgery went well, the aftermath was less smooth. Since this was the second time that Bruce's chest had been opened, the healing process was a lot more difficult. The pain from his surgery was excruciating, and the recovery was slow, but, eventually, Bruce made it out of the hospital. With his LVAD tacked to his side, Sharon took him home where his return was celebrated by his family and two giant dogs.

For once obedient, Bruce completely changed his diet and measured his blood sugar four times a day. Together with Sharon's cooking and his own discipline, Bruce was able to get control of his blood sugar. He worked tirelessly on his stationary bicycle and reported his progress to Dr. Farber at his weekly appointments. He monitored his blood pressure and his resting heart rate. Eventually, he was able to live as normal of a life as he could with the pump implanted in his chest and a machine strapped to his side. Bruce was thankful that he was able to be active, to live, even if it meant being dependent on a machine.

Almost a year after his homecoming, Bruce began to notice a grinding sound. Something inside his chest was making a strange noise, something not right. He called Dr. Farber's office and they made room for him in that afternoon's clinic schedule. He sat on the exam table, afraid to move as Dr. Farber performed electronic testing to detect any problems with the LVAD. Bruce knew she would find something. He knew his device was malfunctioning. He wasn't sure if the grinding was a noise or a feeling, but he was positive it was there when it shouldn't be.

Dr. Farber raised her eyebrows. "It's working just fine, Bruce," she said. "The test doesn't show any abnormalities, and your flows are holding up nicely." She looked at him as he sat, motionless. She hadn't seen him like this before, so alert and so silent. Somehow she knew that the computer must be wrong.

"We'll bring you in," she decided, "and watch you in the hospital overnight."

Bruce nodded and got down from the exam table. He had already packed his bag.

My friend and co-intern, Dr. Jason Tepian, was taking care of Bruce just as things started to go downhill. Jason had met Bruce months before I rotated into the CCU, and he had told me about his sickest patient over coffee breaks and late night calls. Jason was on Bruce's "primary team," which meant he was one of Bruce's daytime interns, the one who wrote the note on the chart every day, who followed every lab value, every fever, every heartbeat. He reported to the attending every day, and together the team developed a plan to help Bruce to see tomorrow.

Jason arrived every morning at 6 a.m. The elevator carried him and his coffee cup to the top floor of the hospital, where he dropped off his bags in the call room and set out down the hall for the CCU. When the sliding doors opened for him, the CCU air would hit him in the face like a wet rag. This was his morning ritual, and every day it was the same thing.

Bruce was in dire straights. He'd been admitted a few weeks earlier after Dr. Farber brought him in for observation, and it hadn't taken long for them to figure out what the problem was. The ball bearings in the LVAD were grinding away and wearing down. The pump was failing. Bruce had become incredibly short of breath, his legs swelled up like balloons, his blood pressure plummeted, and he had been placed on the ventilator, which required a long plastic tube down his vocal cords and into his lungs. It was just a matter of time before the LVAD would fail completely.

Jason wrote his daily progress note meticulously, the same thing every day. The first line would say, "Patient unresponsive and sedated on the ventilator." The next few lines would record Bruce's vital signs and Bruce's painfully unchanging results of the physical exam. Next, he'd move on to the medication list, which easily had twenty different entries. Then, he'd write the medical plan, copying it from the day before, changing it ever so slightly to comment on Bruce's urine output, his white count, and his temperature. He followed the therapeutic drug levels of the medications Bruce was getting, making sure they were at the right dose. Everything had to be completed perfectly by 10 a.m., at which time the attending would come for rounds.

Medically, Bruce was in bad shape. Jason glanced over his notes from the day. He would have to present Bruce's case to Dr. Farber today,

Lauren Van Scoy, M.D.

knowing full well that Dr. Farber knew Bruce's story backward and forward. But the role of the intern is to start with the same old phrase, "This is a 54-year-old man with past medical history of . . .". It was right around the words *past medical history* that Dr. Farber interrupted Jason, anxious to get on with the daily update.

"I know who he is, doctor."

"Oh. Okay, do you not want a formal presentation?" Jason was unsure how to proceed. Some attendings wanted to hear the full report on rounds, and some just wanted to jump to the nitty gritty. Dr. Farber let him know she was more of a nitty-gritty type, and so Jason got to the point.

"His blood pressure has been dangerously low through the night. He hasn't been conscious much and his extremities are cold, so we don't think his circulation is holding up very well," he reported.

The team heard Dr. Farber swear under her breath. Everyone knew what it meant. The LVAD was finally failing. The heart wasn't pumping efficiently enough to keep the blood pressure up, and his organs weren't getting enough oxygen without a strong blood flow. Bruce would have to be switched to a pneumatic driver, which is essentially a hand-crank, compared to the electronic portability of an LVAD. He would have to stay in the hospital until he got a transplant, if an organ became available before Bruce's own heart gave up.

Every day was a new challenge. Jason had to draw blood, and Bruce's poor veins had been stuck a zillion times over. Some of Bruce's medications had to run through a central line, a line that feeds directly into the heart and is placed in through the neck, or near the clavicle, going down into the body about two inches before it feeds directly to the blood vessels leading to the heart. The line is a portal to the bloodstream and also a direct highway for dangerous bacteria to pass through, so it has to be changed frequently to prevent infection. So, about every seven days, Jason inserted a huge needle into Bruce's neck to feed the new line into the heart.

Bruce eventually needed a feeding tube. He remained on the ventilator. He was developing severe weakness and infections from being in the same position for weeks at a time. He required heavy doses of sedatives and pain medications just to keep him comfortable while lying in bed. Medically speaking, he had nothing going for him. Most of the interns privately thought that Dr. Farber should discuss with Bruce's family the possibility of converting Bruce's goals of care from aggressive to palliative care to spare him from the pain and medical torture we were imposing.

Since I was the night intern taking care of Bruce, Jason would give me daily updates about all the horrors Bruce was enduring, and we had many discussions about the fact that Bruce's situation made him an appropriate candidate for hospice care, a service whose primary objective is to make patients comfortable and give them a chance for dignity and peace when death becomes inevitable. The prolonged suffering seemed to only highlight the fact that Bruce was dying, Jason explained and I saw for myself as I performed my nightly exams in Bruce's isolation room. Jason and I also talked about Sharon, and how the months of agony seemed to be more than any one woman could take, but she continued to have hope when no one else seemed to. No one except Dr. Farber.

And then, it happened. One afternoon, Bruce's heart sighed and gave up. The nurse yelled out in panic when she saw the monitor. Within a second, the crash cart was there and Jason began CPR. Fifteen people careened into the room all at once and the "code" began. The intensity level ramped up; where there had once been the quiet buzzing of machines and soft beeps, there were now loud noises, shouting, and chaos.

Jason's muscular arms could hardly compress Bruce's massive chest. He had to push against the chest wall hard enough so that the force of his hands would pump his heart. Bruce was already on the ventilator, so his lungs were taken care of. But they had to restart the heart.

"Epi!" the cardiology fellow yelled as he came sprinting into the room. Lucky for Jason, the fellow had been nearby. The fellow was a lot more senior than Jason, and Jason was relieved to hear the fellow's voice calling for epinephrine. Jason didn't look up from the CPR. Sweat was dripping from his brow by this point, and he didn't know what was happening around him, but he knew he had to keep the compressions going. He had to pump Bruce's heart.

"This is it," thought Jason. "No way will he come out of this."

But the code continued. The nurses skillfully obtained the blood samples. The fellow was masterfully running the code from the foot of the bed and the noise level was increasing exponentially. Jason looked up to catch a glance of the heart rhythm on the monitor.

"Hold CPR!" the fellow yelled above the chaos. Jason stopped, grateful for the rest.

"Check pulse!" was the next command. The monitor showed a flat line.

"No pulse!" a nurse responded from deep within the swarm of people working on Bruce.

"Continue CPR!" said the fellow. "And give atropine!"

And so it went for two more minutes. CPR continued. The IV bicarbonate went in, followed by the IV calcium. The nurses were scurrying around, carrying out the orders as the cardiology fellow shouted them out. By now the medical students had all come in to catch some of the action. The eager ones stood behind Jason waiting for their chance to do *real* CPR. And they each had their chance. Jason and the students took turns compressing Bruce's chest.

"Hold CPR! Check pulse!" yelled the fellow. The medical student froze, not moving his hands out of CPR position.

"I have a pulse," said the nurse.

Jason's eyes shot to the monitor. He had a rhythm! Jason looked to the fellow, who despite it all was stoic and calm. He's got a pulse. He's got a rhythm. He's back from the dead.

Now what?

A little over a year later, I was back on rotation in the CCU, this time as a senior resident in charge of an intern. I printed out my patient list, and right at the top was Bruce's name. Apparently, he was alive. I couldn't believe it. Had he been here this whole time? I could only imagine the state he must be in after all this time. I had heard about the code, but not much else. His chart must be on its hundredth volume, I thought. Starting a new rotation with all new patients can be daunting, especially when one of those patients has had a long, complicated course like Bruce. It's easier, sometimes, just to head into the room and start there, see what you've got, rather than paging through the unending pages of a very long chart. So I didn't bother to look in the chart; I needed to see *this* with my own eyes first.

I stopped outside his room at the isolation cart and gowned up with the familiar yellow garb. *The Infection*, I remembered. I stepped into the room and almost fell over.

"Hiya, doc!" Bruce said. He was sitting in a chair next to the window, eating breakfast and watching his television.

"Uh, hi," I said cautiously. "Are you Mr. Sellers?"

"The one and only," he responded.

I squinted my eyes to see more closely. It *was* him. Instead of a horizontal patient, here was a man sitting upright in a chair. He was strikingly tall and muscular, wearing a Harley Davidson t-shirt, which was quite a contrast to my five foot nothing, petite self. He had the typical biker look to him, with brown eyes that were gentle yet fierce. Replacing the ventilator tube that had been in his mouth was a smile that went from ear to ear. If you saw him on the street, you might think he was surly, but up close, he was a gentle giant. I couldn't believe that this was the man beneath the machines.

"You probably don't remember me, but I'm Dr. Van Scoy. I took care of you a year ago when you were, uh . . .". I hesitated, not knowing quite how to say the words.

"Out of it?" Bruce finished for me.

"Yeah. Out of it." I was kicking myself for not having read the chart before I'd walked in the room. I had no idea what was going on, and I had no idea where to take the conversation next. I wasn't ready to do an evaluation on *this* person named Bruce; I had expected to see a comatose patient, the Bruce I remembered. So I bailed out the way most residents do when they get into a situation where they don't quite know what to say: I plucked my pager off my hip and said, "Hang on, this thing is vibrating. I gotta go answer this. I'll be back."

"I'll be here!" Bruce spooned some eggs into his mouth.

I made a beeline for his chart. I flipped it open and paged to the most recent progress note. "Healed sternal wound post transplant." No fever. No white count. No bacteria. No vac. The infection had actually cleared.

My first reaction was shock and then an overwhelming guilt coursed through me. I had written him off as dead. I thought back to my feelings of how *cruel* it seemed that we were keeping Bruce alive in such a state of obvious suffering. I'd thought that he had no chance for recovery. That he was a goner and we were wasting precious medical resources on a patient who had no chance for survival. I'd wanted to forego CPR and not resuscitate this man's crippled heart. I'd thought for sure our medical interventions would be all for naught. But now, he was eating breakfast.

Suddenly, everything I thought I understood about critical care was wrong and flipped upside down. I'd felt disgusted by how aggressive we'd been with Bruce's care way back when. Hadn't Jason and I talked about the fact that this patient was clearly not going to recover, that he clearly should be a DNR ("do not resuscitate")? And then, he had coded! And they had saved him. Why, I wondered back then? For what? And now, it was very clear to me what we had saved him for: so that he could survive.

The revelation was terrifying, and being fresh out of medical school with little experience in matters of life and death, I immediately jumped to all the wrong conclusions. I assumed I was a horrible doctor. I worried that I'd never be able to face families looking to me for guidance about their loved one's end-of-life care in light of life's uncertainties.

I brought my woes and worries to my mentor, Dr. Poe, an intensive care physician I had bonded with early on in my medical training.

"You're not a terrible physician," he reassured me, "and you certainly weren't wrong in thinking that Bruce may have been better off with less invasive measures and comfort care." He paused, and my puzzled look prompted him to continue.

He explained that a do-not-resuscitate order would have been a perfectly reasonable decision for his family to make, or for a physician to advise, given his overall condition. Shifting the focus of his care to comfort measures would have been reasonable, too. Our job as physicians isn't to predict the future, but to guide our patients' families so they know what to expect with whatever route they choose to pursue, whether that be aggressive care or less so. Some people would never want to experience the things Bruce experienced, even if it meant living longer.

"Recovery doesn't happen overnight," Dr. Poe observed, "and I bet that in the time since you saw this patient last, he's been through hell and back. You have to wonder what the cost was for him, physically and emotionally. What has he gone through since then and what kind of quality of life does he have today?"

"He's alive, isn't he?" Angry at myself, I sounded accusatory. "What if we hadn't tried resuscitating him back then?" My confusion was making me defensive, and my guilt made me want Dr. Poe to scold me harshly, telling me that my clinical judgement was way off base.

"There's no right or wrong in these matters, L. J.," he said softly. "There is only choice."

Three days later, I strolled into Bruce's room. It had taken me several days to figure out exactly what had happened to him during the last year. I'd read his chart from cover to cover, shaking my head in disbelief. After his code, he'd been stabilized and switched onto the pneumatic driver, the hand-pump of LVADs. He'd been plugged into that wall for many months, only able to walk around the side of his bed, let alone get outside and enjoy a breath of fresh air. Yet his heart continued to beat, and with each beat, he grew a tiny bit stronger.

One spectacular night, the call had come in. A heart was available. The surgeon popped his head into Bruce's hospital room and said the magic words: "Guess what?!!"

Bruce recalled for me later the moment when he realized that he was getting a heart, and he insisted on doing one thing and one thing only: he would walk down to the operating room. The nurses tried to coax him onto the gurney, or at least into a wheelchair, but Bruce the Rebel knew that he could walk, so he walked his way right down into the OR with his surgeon by his side, awaiting the chance to open his chest for a third time in order to place the healthy heart. But after the third open-heart surgery, Bruce's sternum was angry, and Bruce's body could not fight off the infection. His sternal wound took over eight months to heal, and the infection ate away at his chest wall. He endured eight months of dressing changes and antibiotics, of sedatives and pain medications, and against all odds, he beat The Infection again and finally began the long and tedious road to rehabilitation.

"G'mornin!" I said. I was in a surprisingly good mood after reading Bruce's amazing chart.

A single large tear dripped from Bruce's eyes, salting my good mood. Had he been a little old lady having a cry, I would have sat on the edge of her bed and taken her hand, or perhaps placed my own hand on her shoulder to inquire what was wrong. Instead, I stood frozen and silent, caught off guard.

I quickly gathered my composure. "What's wrong?"

Bruce pulled himself together in a way that only a man can do and answered, "I just found out information about my donor."

I kept quiet, waiting for him to continue on his own.

The Gift of Life, the organ donation agency, doesn't share personal information between donors and recipients unless both families agree, and even then, they divulge information very slowly. They have to be sensitive to both sides because after all, for every recipient saved, a donor must die.

"He was a biker," sniffed Bruce. "He died in a motorcycle accident."

I didn't know what to say. I had heard about the so-called "biker brotherhood," but to see Bruce sobbing like this, I didn't know how to comfort him, so I reverted to my textbook training: .

"Wow." I said. "How do you feel about that?" An open-ended question is supposed to elicit the patient's emotions. I didn't know if the technique would work on Bruce the Biker. But it did.

"I don't know, doc," he said. "I don't know. After everything I've been through, I don't even know how to thank him. All I do know is that as soon as I get out of here, I'm going to get on my bike, I'm gonna rev it hard, and I know I'm going to feel my heart smile."

* * *

When I first met Bruce, I was in my earliest years as a physician, an intern without the experience yet to accurately predict which patients were highly likely to die, and which ones might not. At that time, I didn't understand why Bruce was one of the few who had a chance.

When I'd see Bruce in the unit at night, I'd see a patient with a lot of things attached to him—a ventilator, medications, a vac dressing—and compare him to all the other patients I'd seen in similar or less severe conditions. Patients who had died. I foresaw a similar outcome in his case.

What I didn't see back then was the potential for Bruce's healthy body to recover. I saw a man suffering under the assault from modern medicine's best intentions, and I felt an instinct to try and ease his suffering. I couldn't understand Dr. Farber's optimism, and I couldn't help but wonder why, after Bruce's cardiac arrest, she had not recommended to his wife and family that comfort measures be considered. I never asked Dr. Farber if she had considered making a recommendation toward DNR, but in retrospect, I would guess that her answer would have been no, simply because Bruce had a chance of survival, a chance to recover. Most important, he also had the ability.

Other than his heart disease, Bruce was healthy. Compared to most patients in the ICU, he was young and strong. He was forty-nine years old with no other major medical problems other than his diabetes and heart failure. He was not a geriatric patient living in a nursing home with limited ability to move around or without mental capacity. Instead, he was fully functional other than his heart disease, and he had the ability and family support to comply with the vigorous demands of his recovery. He was able to exercise and work toward regaining muscle mass and reversing the muscle atrophy he developed during his weeks on life support. He had been well enough before his illness that he could and would survive.

Ever since Bruce granted me the interview allowing me to write his incredible story, we've stayed in touch, and although I wish it weren't so, Bruce didn't ride his motorcycle off into the sunset. In fact, he hasn't even sat on a motorcycle since his release from the hospital. He is admitted to the hospital often and when he is, he sends a message to me in some way or another, inviting me to stop by and say hello. I've seen Bruce struggle with more infections, complications from his wounds and medications, and from the frustration and depression of being hospitalized frequently and often. Bruce's recovery, although miraculous, changed his life forever in a way that I couldn't then imagine, nor do I underestimate now.

Each time Bruce and I meet, I learn something new about survivors of critical illness. He shows me that for every patient we can't save, there is always a patient we *can* save. Sorting out who is who is part of which group makes our job as critical care doctors unique. With such uncertainty in matters of life and death, you might consider the obvious question: how can anyone know when there is no chance of recovery? When can you really know when enough is enough? Sadly, there is no easy answer and certainly no magic cure for those who have a chance.

The only thing we can promise is to try to reverse what's reversible in hopes of establishing a meaningful recovery. What defines a truly meaningful recovery is different for each of us..

Discussion Questions

1. Bruce was in a state of near death for many months and endured many invasive procedures prior to getting his heart transplant. What were the trade-offs for Bruce and his family as they continued full aggressive medical therapy? What sacrifices did he make in order to survive his illness?

2. Bruce was a middle aged, strong and healthy man prior to his life threatening illness. Consider how a person's condition prior to serious illness influences their ability to recover. How should this impact decisions made about invasive and aggressive medical interventions?

3. What would you be willing to give up in order to survive a life-threatening illness (discomfort, independence, ability to eat, walk, etc)? What would you not be willing to sacrifice?

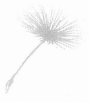

2

Breathless

No matter how much I love my work, Monday mornings always seem to be a kick in the teeth. This one in particular wasn't starting well at all. Having trudged in from the rainy day outside, my socks and ankles were cold and wet from the cuffs of my scrubs dragging through puddles on the Philadelphia streets. Even though I had been off for the entire weekend, a rarity for me, I still had the feeling of exhaustion soaking into my bones. I'd woken up early, feeling anxious about returning to the hospital, I would certainly be getting many new patients who'd come in over the weekend, so I had a lot of catching up to do. Since four in the morning, my mind had been racing with questions left over from Friday.

What did Mr. Smith's CT scan show? Did Mrs. Cane's renal function improve over the weekend? And what about Mrs. Shaney's abdominal surgery? Did her family make it to the hospital in time to wish her well before she was whisked off to the OR? As I dropped my bag in my locker, I stopped myself from logging into the computer in the physician's lounge to get answers. Instead, I decided my first stop would have to be the cafeteria. I needed coffee in a wicked way. No time even to print my patient list. I had a lot of catching up to do on the weekend's happenings, and I needed a caffeine fix to prepare me for my Monday morning.

The elevator opened with a "ding" and I stepped inside a car already packed with nurses, doctors, and students, all heading for their own morning buzz. We stood in silence and descended to the second floor.

The first to get out, I quickened my pace to beat the masses to the coffee shop, and, of course, my beeper went off. *Nothing worse than getting paged before your day's even started*, I thought. Stopping at the house phone on the wall, I watched as all the others passed me to get into the coffee line. I dialled the number and waited.

"Seventeenth floor," a voice answered.

"Hi, this is Dr. Van Scoy. I'm returning a page."

"Hi L. J. It's Kevin!" a voice chirped. Kevin was one of the medical students rounding with me this month. Glad that it wasn't an emergency, I sighed in relief, although I was somewhat irritated that I was missing my prime spot in the coffee line.

"Hi, Kevin, what's up?"

"I wanted to let you know that Mr. Smith's CT scan was normal and I already printed your patient list," he told me.

I smiled. Things were looking up. Kevin had just saved me from fighting the other doctors for computer time. "Thanks, Kevin. I'm gonna grab a cup of coffee and I'll meet you guys up on the seventeenth, okay? Want a cup?"

"I already got mine, thanks," he said. "One of the nurses asked me if I could have you see Mrs. Chandler in room 1772 first, because she needs more pain medication. I'll check it out, and I'll see you up here!"

"On my way. Thanks, Kevin," I answered.

After hanging up the phone, I stepped into the coffee line, no longer concerned about the long wait. Having Kevin on the team was a true asset since he was eager and motivated, and I knew he'd be able to help me make up the lost time. By the time I got out of the elevator on the seventeenth floor, I felt like a new person.

"I saw Mrs. Chandler already!" Kevin called as he saw me coming down the hall. "I can tell you about her to you, if you want."

One advantage of a good student is that they typically pore through the charts and can present a succinct story. Sipping from my cup, I nodded to Kevin to proceed.

"Okay, Mrs. Chandler is eighty-eight years old and has lung cancer. It's spread to her bones, all along her spine," he began. "Apparently, she was here a few weeks ago with pneumonia and has been admitted at least a dozen times in the last year for different infections and episodes of back pain."

A familiar story: lung cancer is a beast when it spreads to the bones. It causes tremendous back and bone pain, so if what Kevin was reporting was correct, then reigning in Mrs. Chandler's pain would be a real challenge.

"All right." I waved him ahead of me. "Let's go see her together."

Kevin led the way to Mrs. Chandler's room while I drained the last of my coffee and tossed the cup in the trash as we entered. A thin, frail woman lay before me on the hospital bed.

She seemed to be swallowed by a sea of white hospital blankets, as only her head popped out above the covers. She had prominent cheekbones, probably because her facial muscles were wasting away, and her eyes were dark against her pale skin. From the look on her face and the agony in her eyes, I could tell that her pain was deep and raw. At her bedside table was her untouched breakfast tray.

After I introduced myself, Mrs. Chandler only moaned.

I continued, "This is Kevin, a medical student working with me. Together, we work with Dr. Simmons, who is your attending, or lead physician, and we will be the team taking care of you here in the hospital."

"I need pain meds," she moaned, clearly not interested in my formalities.

"I'll check to see when the nurse last gave you your medication, and if it's time for more, I'll have her bring it to you. Have you eaten anything today?" I asked.

"No, too much pain," she answered.

"Okay, tell me where it hurts." Gently, I sat on the edge of the bed.

"All over. I need pain meds!" Clearly, she was not keen on answering my questions, and I couldn't blame her.

Kevin shrugged. Apparently, he hadn't been able to glean much information from her either.

Just then, someone else came crashing into the room, shouting as she threw down her jacket and purse. "She needs her pain meds, miss!" Raindrops lined her coat, and I guessed that she had just arrived at the hospital.

"I'm sorry, but we haven't met. I'm Dr. Van Scoy. Who are you?" Maybe being polite would hide my defensiveness.

"I'm Lisa, her daughter. Are you gonna just let my mother lie here in pain like that?"

Inwardly, I cringed at the accusation, but I calmly told her I would go get the nurse so that her mother could have some more morphine.

"Morphine doesn't help her pain." Lisa was even angrier now.

"I understand. I've only just met your mom, and I need to review her chart to get familiar with what medication will be best for her, and I'll speak with Dr. Simmons, her attending physician, about changing her pain regimen. I'll be back with Dr. Simmons in a little bit." I gave Kevin the "let's go" look and left the room, annoyed that I had to abort the initial interview and physical exam.

It was obvious that having Lisa present for any further conversation with Mrs. Chandler would be counterproductive, as Lisa was already quite angry and I simply didn't have enough information to defuse the tension. I hoped we could talk more with Mrs. Chandler herself once the pain medicine was administered, and perhaps by then Lisa would be less tense. I'd send Kevin back once Lisa was settled and while I tried to get some information from the chart. He would love the opportunity to shine, and I decided to let him have his chance.

Three days later, while I was sitting at the nurse's station reviewing the daily labs for my patients, disgruntled voices erupted nearby, and I glanced up from my computer to see Lisa gesticulating at the floor clerk. It was the same scene I'd witnessed every few hours over the last several days. Lisa was irate and insistent because the latest dose of her mother's pain medication was three minutes late.

When Mrs. Chandler's nurse for the day came within earshot, I asked her how we were doing with managing Mrs. Chandler's pain. Jenny had a much better understanding of pain levels than I did, and I trusted her assessments. She was in a patient's room many times a day, whereas I would usually visit only for rounds or if there was a new problem.

Jenny told me that the night team had changed Mrs. Chandler's medication to Dilaudid, and she was administering it every four hours. "I think she's fine now. When I turn her she has some pain, but overall, I think the Dilaudid is working much better than the morphine did."

Even though I was relieved to hear that, I knew it meant I'd have to go in and calm Lisa down. If her mother's pain was well controlled, there'd be no benefit from more narcotics. Walking to the room, I contemplated how I'd talk with Lisa and what to say, trying to remind myself that her aggressive behavior likely had very little to do with me or the medical team, and more to do with the cancer claiming her mother's life.

Lisa was trying to restore her mother to the woman she knew and so dearly missed. Yet Mrs. Chandler had cancer in her bones, and she would probably never be pain-free. I tried to imagine, and accept, Lisa's outrage. She couldn't make demands on her mother's tumor, so instead, she made demands upon the medical team. Interactions with Lisa could be infuriating, but accepting them and embracing the place from which they came was the least we could do.

Mrs. Chandler's primary physician, Dr. Sara Simmons, Kevin, and I had had daily discussions with Lisa about Mrs. Chandler's grim prognosis and our continued efforts at pain control. Every day, we'd given Lisa updates, but none offered much hope that the cancer's progression could be halted or even slowed. We'd raised the possibility of palliative or hospice care, which would focus on making Mrs. Chandler's symptom management and pain control the main priority knowing further medical treatments seemed unlikely to be beneficial. We could focus on keeping Mrs. Chandler as pain-free as possible, we'd suggested, but Lisa had refused to consider it.

Instead, she wanted and expected the impossible, a return to her mom's pain-free, cancer-free life. Unfortunately, we simply couldn't give her that.

As I approached the room, I hoped that perhaps today Lisa would open her mind to the idea of palliation, but realistically, I knew I was better off preparing myself for the onslaught.

Mrs. Chandler was alone in her room. She lay in her bed, her mouth wide open and her eyes rolled up into her head. She looked dead, and a shot of panic jolted through my body. My eyes darted to her chest to confirm she was breathing, and I saw that her respirations were unnaturally slow. She looked groggy, but one thing was certain, she wasn't in extreme pain. I heard the toilet flush in Mrs. Chandler's bathroom, and Lisa joined me at the bedside.

"Look at her!" Lisa exclaimed. "She looks awful! She's in pain! What are you going to do to fix this?"

"Lisa, your mom isn't in pain right now. She's dying from her cancer."

As Lisa's jaw began to twitch with building anger, I held up my hand then pointed to the monitor. "Her heart rate is normal. That's a reassuring sign that she's not in pain. If she was, her heart rate would probably be much higher. We're giving her the medicine she needs already, and adding even more sedation isn't going to make her better. In fact, it will make her worse, and she could end up on the breathing machine. What we're trying to achieve is a level of pain control that enables her to be comfortable yet more alert and interactive. It's important that we don't under treat her pain, but it's equally important that we don't over treat her."

"I'm calling Dr. Simmons, then, if you won't give her any more pain meds." Calling my attending was a trick she had learned recently as a way to punish me when I didn't do what she wanted.

"No problem. In fact, I'll go get her." I left the room, happy for the excuse to go.

Lisa was nodding enthusiastically as Dr. Simmons explained our new plan: an epidural. Not a cure, but a long-term option for pain control that would allow us to decrease the amount of narcotics and enable Mrs. Chandler to wake up a little and be more interactive. Lisa was clutching her hands together in excitement as Dr. Simmons explained the procedure. Mrs. Chandler was feebly nodding in agreement.

The following day, we consulted the anesthesiologists to place the epidural, and we began to reduce the narcotics. Everyone was on the same page. We had found a way to satisfy Lisa and, more important, we had a solid plan on how to deal with Mrs. Chandler's pain in a way that wouldn't over sedate her. I only hoped it would work. Time would tell, as it can be a few days before an epidural takes full effect. If it worked, we could start the process of getting Mrs. Chandler ready for gentle rehab. I'd have Kevin call the physical therapists first thing in the morning. Maybe we could gain Lisa's trust, too.

When I hit the floor the next morning, Kevin was urgent. "L. J., can you come look at Mrs. Chandler?" His voice sounded shaky. I wasn't alarmed, though, as Kevin was a bit of an over-reactor.

"Sure, what's up?"

"She's not looking good: her oxygen levels are dropping."

"Okay, let's go see her."

As we walked, Kevin filled me in on the evening's events. "She had a few episodes of low oxygen levels overnight, and they had to put on an oxygen mask for a brief time."

Now this was worrisome. "All right, let's order a chest X-ray and go get a blood gas kit."

As he obediently headed for the medical supply room, I tried to formulate a quick list of possible causes for Mrs. Chandler's rapid drop in oxygen. Could she have a blood clot in her lung? Could she have fluid building up in or around her lungs? Or perhaps it was as simple as mucus plugging up some of the airway? Or could this just be a natural decline from her lung cancer?

When I reached the room, Mrs. Chandler's breathing was labored, and her oxygen level was flashing a mere 81 percent on the monitor. If I couldn't fix her oxygen level quickly, I would need to intubate her, place a tube into her lungs so she could be started on a breathing machine, and begin full-fledged life support. I desperately wanted to avoid that because it would probably result in even more suffering for Mrs. Chandler.

Jenny was in the process of turning up the oxygen flow rate on the wall meter, and I saw that as she did so, the oxygen level rose to 94 percent within a few breaths. Encouraging! As I approached Mrs. Chandler, I called to her, and she barely opened her eyes. A quick physical exam told me her heart was beating quickly; otherwise, it sounded relatively normal.

With surprisingly little effort, Jenny was able to lift Mrs. Chandler forward so I could listen to her lungs: soft crackles. Tapping on Mrs. Chandler's back, I could hear a dullness that suggested fluid might be building up around her lungs. Her blood pressure was 130/80, which meant we could try using medications to decrease the amount of fluid in and around her lung without bottoming out her blood pressure.

"Let's give her some Lasix, Jenny, and we can shut off her IV fluids for now. Maybe she is just a little fluid overloaded."

Jenny nodded in agreement, and Kevin came into the room.

"Here's the blood gas kit," he offered.

"Go ahead." I motioned to Mrs. Chandler's arm. "You do it."

Kevin smiled and began the process of cleaning Mrs. Chandler's arm and looking for his point of entry to draw blood. The test would give us information about Mrs. Chandler's ventilation status, as well as her oxygen level. I was hoping that the diuretic I had just ordered and the increase in the oxygen flow rate would stabilize her long enough for us to figure out exactly what was causing her decline.

Mrs. Chandler flinched appropriately as Kevin stuck her arm with the needle, a good sign that she was becoming more responsive with the increase in her oxygen level.

"Are you feeling any better?" I asked Mrs. Chandler, whose eyes were now more alert, and she seemed to be perking up. Her oxygen level now read 100%.

"I guess so," she answered feebly. "I feel okay."

"Vitals every five minutes until we figure this out," I instructed the nurse and as I left the room I added, "Stay with her, Kevin. I'll be back in a few minutes." Even though the immediate crisis had been averted, I knew we weren't out of the woods.

A few hours later, we were worse off than when we had started. Mrs. Chandler's oxygen requirements had escalated to a full 100 percent non-rebreather facemask. This was the maximum amount of oxygen we could administer without a ventilator, and it meant Mrs. Chandler would have to be transferred to the intensive care unit. The chest X-ray had confirmed that fluid surrounded her lung and revealed a large pleural effusion that would probably need to be drained. The diuretic had increased Mrs. Chandler's urination enough to dry out the insides of her lungs somewhat, but the fluid building up around the lung was a more pressing problem. To drain it, we would have to perform a thoracentesis, or a "tap," where we'd place a needle into her back between her ribs, just far enough to draw the fluid out of the sac surrounding her lungs.

"Kevin," I said, "give Lisa a call." It was surprising that Lisa hadn't visited yet today, anyway. "Let her know her mother is taking a turn for the worse and she should come to the hospital."

Kevin's eyes widened as he realized what I was saying. He was bright. He understood Mrs. Chandler was about to develop respiratory failure and that she would require the ventilator by the time the day was out. I gritted my teeth as I thought about the cancer load in Mrs. Chandler's lungs. If we put her on the ventilator, it would be nearly impossible to get her off again. Things were about to get a whole lot worse.

Dr. Simmons was yelling at me over the phone: "Do NOT intubate this woman!"

She knew as well as I did what the outcome of this would be, but what choice did we have? We did not have an advance directive or living will, and Mrs. Chandler was too sick to tell me what her wishes were and had never really given us a clear answer about how she wanted to treat her cancer. Comfort care was the most medically sound treatment for someone as seriously ill and in as much pain as Mrs. Chandler. As I saw it, my job was to get Lisa to understand that her mom was dreadfully sick and that putting her on the ventilator was essentially the definition of finality. I had to go in armed with information, so I went to the break room to get a cup of coffee and gather my thoughts. Exhausted and worried, I plopped myself down at the table and drummed my fingers against its surface as I reviewed the facts.

Mrs. Chandler had an enormous amount of tumor in her lungs. It had spread to her bones and was eroding her spine, causing tremendous pain. Chemotherapy and radiation had not worked. Her labored breathing was not solely because of the fluid, but it was also the inevitable progression of her disease. Her old X-rays showed a pattern of frequent pneumonias and fluid build-ups. Her lungs were tiring out and, despite all her previous "recoveries" from similar episodes, it was just too much. Cancer was coming to claim Mrs. Chandler.

Could I get Lisa to understand that putting her mother on the ventilator was not a good option? Mrs. Chandler's breathing problems were not temporary. Even if we removed the fluid, the amount of cancer in the lung made it highly unlikely that she would ever be weaned off the ventilator.

Out of the corner of my eye, I saw Kevin hang up the phone. He nodded at me, telling me that Lisa was on her way.

As expected, when Lisa arrived, she was livid. "What did you do? You put that epidural in and now she's not breathing! You need to FIX this! You need to fix my mom!"

My blood boiled. I couldn't fix cancer. Feeling angry, helpless, frustrated, and defeated, I didn't want to have this conversation starting with this tone, but I didn't have much of a choice.

"Lisa, please calm down. Let's talk about what's happening and we can talk about what we're going to have to do next, okay?" I was practically pleading with her. Placing my hand on Mrs. Chandler's leg, I tried to convey to Lisa how much I truly cared about what happened to her mother. "First of all, I don't think your mom's deterioration is due to the epidural or even the narcotics we're giving her."

Lisa shot upright in her chair, ready to let loose a mouthful, but I held up my hand to stop her.

"She has some fluid building up in her lungs as a result of her cancer. And even though we can remove the fluid with a needle to try and temporize her situation, this is really the cancer taking its toll on her lungs."

"I don't want to hear about cancer," Lisa said. "I want you to fix my mom!"

"Lisa, I'm trying to tell you I can't fix your mom. She is dying of cancer." Lisa was in denial and grieving, but I had to maintain my composure and not avoid the truth.

The conversation went around in circles for a few minutes until it was apparent I needed a new approach, so I took her out to the nurse's station. Together, we crossed the invisible "no patients" line behind the main desk, and I pulled up the film. The whited-out lung glowed. Lisa shrugged her shoulders.

"So?"

"So, *this*." I pointed to the whited-out lung. "This is what is making her short of breath. Not simply pain or the epidural. Pain doesn't do *this*." My finger poked the screen.

"She was breathing yesterday! Does cancer happen overnight? No! It was something you did that stopped her from breathing."

"You're right, cancer doesn't happen overnight, but eventually, the disease progresses. All the evidence we have right now tells us that the disease is progressing, and she has reached that critical point where her lungs can't take much more. There's always a time when patients with end-stage cancer deteriorate, and I think this is what is happening to your mom."

Lisa unloaded a stream of profanity. Her body began to sway from side to side as she shifted her weight. I was afraid Lisa was going to become violent.

Taking a step back, I asked her to leave the nurses' station. Showing her the X-ray had been completely ineffective, so I had to retreat. Lisa stormed off in a huff back to her mom's room, and Kevin took his place at my side.

"That's how you do it," I said sarcastically. "I hope you were taking notes."

Back at Mrs. Chandler's bedside, the nurses were watching her oxygen levels drop again. Kevin came to retrieve me from the nurses' station, where I had remained since the confrontation with Lisa as I tried to facilitate moving Mrs. Chandler to the intensive care unit.

"They need you again," he said. "She's breathing at a rate of thirty-five." Normal is fourteen.

Now Mrs. Chandler was too unstable to attempt doing the tap, which I had hoped might give her some relief. She would probably need a pressure mask, called a "bipap," which fits tightly and connects to a machine that pushes air under pressure into the lungs. It's a form of mechanical ventilation without using a tube that goes in the throat. It might help decrease the work of breathing on Mrs. Chandler's already weak muscles, but would also be incredibly uncomfortable for her, having air forced into her lungs.

When I saw her, Mrs. Chandler was gasping, and it was clear that the bipap wasn't going to be enough. If we were going to resuscitate Mrs. Chandler, it was time to put her on the ventilator. Lisa was on her cell phone, pacing on the other side of the room as the nurses were working to place a new oxygen mask.

"Seventeenth floor," she said into the phone. "Turn right off the elevator and she's in room 1772. The doctor is here."

I looked into Mrs. Chandler's eyes and saw she was lucid.

"Mrs. Chandler, I'm right here. Listen, I need you to tell me if you want me to put you on a machine to help you breathe," I said. She clutched my hand. "Lisa is here, too," I said, hoping the comment would soften Lisa up a little. "Do you want me to do that? Are you willing to be on life support?"

She looked up at me but said nothing.

"My brother is coming," Lisa said. "He'll be here in a minute. He's on the elevator."

Why didn't I know there was a brother? I scolded myself for not having asked about other family members and for assuming Lisa was the only one.

Lisa leaned down to her mother's ear. "Sam is coming, Mom."

In the meantime, I ordered a few more labs and helped the nurses administer medications. Soon, Sam arrived. He entered the room and ran over to his mother. He commented on how thin their mom was to Lisa, and when Sam turned to me, he seemed stoic and calm, a real contrast to his sister, and my heart flooded with hope that he could help us to set the situation right. Sam heard his mother's story and my explanations, nodding his head as I spoke, and he didn't interrupt. He asked me a few pointed questions about the epidural and other medications. Then he pressed his lips together in thought.

Prompting him, I offered, "So, you and Lisa will have to make a decision about where we go from here. Do you know what your mom would have wanted regarding being put on life support?"

Lisa rushed to be first to answer: "Mom wants to live!"

Sam ignored her. "When we brought my mother to the emergency room, the doctors down there asked her what she would want if her heart were to stop, whether she'd want to be resuscitated? Her answer was yes," he remembered aloud.

"That's right!" Lisa seemed lifted to have his support.

Slowly, I offered more for him to consider. "Okay. We want to respect her wishes, and we can put her on the ventilator. But I want you to understand that because her cancer is end stage and so severe, it's unlikely that she will ever get off the ventilator once we put her on it. And it isn't going to fix her underlying problem."

Lisa still wasn't hearing me. "She just needs it to rest for a few hours and then you can take it off."

Sam looked at me as if to ask if that was a possibility.

"Well, it doesn't really work that way," I replied. "Your mom's lungs would be dependent on the ventilator, and although I can't say for certain that she would *never* get off the ventilator, I think it's a real possibility, and I just want you to understand that. Your mom is dying, and we're at the point now where the decisions you make are going to determine the *way* she dies, not *whether* or not she dies."

"Get the machine," Lisa demanded.

Sam went to his mom. "Mom, do you want the breathing machine? Do you?"

Mrs. Chandler didn't respond with anything other than a few sobs. I watched as her heart rate rose, and I decided to call for an anesthesiologist who would perform the intubation, since once the decision was made, we wouldn't have a lot of time.

Sam took Lisa's hand. "Let's talk outside."

I was happy to hear that. I thought for sure Sam was foreseeing the complications of putting Mrs. Chandler on a breathing machine. A tube in the throat. A medically induced coma. The increased possibility of pneumonia. The intensity of the critical care unit. Sam seemed to understand that there wasn't a cure for cancer in the ventilator. He would be the voice of reason, I thought. I had gotten through to him. He would help unite us all so we could move forward in caring for Mrs. Chandler in the most humane way possible. Perhaps he could help me convince Lisa that the breathing machine would only make matters worse.

After a few minutes, they returned and Sam had a look of peace on his face. They had made a decision.

"Put the tube in," he said plainly, his arm around Lisa. Seeing them united in a decision, even a decision I completely disagreed with, made me happy to oblige.

Dr. Roberts, Mrs. Chandler's pulmonary and critical care doctor, got the update an hour after I intubated Mrs. Chandler. He was lying in his bed and reading yesterday's paper when his phone rang. As he listened to the story, his years of experience told him what sort of mess was about to unfurl. He had been following Mrs. Chandler for her chronic shortness of breath, helping to make recommendations to ease the symptoms resulting from the tumors in her lungs. But now, it was another story. Lines, tubes, antibiotics, transfusions, infections, bleeds. She would get them all, he anticipated.

Dr. Roberts had come to accept death as a part of life, but it was the *way* she was going to die that bothered him. Because the family had indicated that they wanted everything done to keep her alive, she was about to become a body supported by machines. The cancer wouldn't stop her heart completely, and the ventilator would do her breathing for her. If her kidneys failed, they would start dialysis. Modern medicine has the ability to do amazing things. We can keep people alive for extraordinary periods of time, but it always left Dr. Roberts wondering: just because we *can* do something, does it mean that we *should?* There wasn't much of a choice in Mrs. Chandler's case, however; she had voiced her wish in the emergency room to be resuscitated, and her next of kin were requesting full and aggressive care. He listened as he heard the plan, muttered a few "uh-huhs" in agreement, hung up the phone, and let out a heavy sigh. Tomorrow was another day. Maybe the family would come around and realize that life support was not a good solution for someone with a terminal disease like cancer. Maybe. But if not, he had an arsenal of modern medicine, perched and ready to perform its "magic."

He thought back to his first meeting with Mrs. Chandler three months before. He'd been consulted by Dr. Simmons to offer specialty care, and at that time, her cancer had caused significant amounts of pleural effusion, or fluid build-up, surrounding the lungs. She'd had a terrible functional status even then, being unable to walk or even sit up without terrible pain and shortness of breath. To remove the fluid, he'd performed a thoracentesis, or tap. Once the fluid was gone, Mrs. Chandler had felt significantly better, but it was only a small victory against her deadly disease. Lisa and Sam adored him for it, and their confidence in Dr. Roberts had been sky-high.

"You really did it, Dr. Roberts!" Lisa had said, snatching him into a huge hug. "You cured her effusions!" Dr. Roberts had been very uncomfortable with her choice of words, as *cure* was not one he would use in the context of Mrs. Chandler. These kinds of effusions always came back, especially when they were caused by cancer.

Despite her best efforts, Dr. Simmons' lengthy discussions with Mrs. Chandler and Lisa hadn't made much of an impact in encouraging them to discuss Mrs. Chandler's end of life wishes. It was a topic they simply couldn't or wouldn't face. Dr. Simmons had described the grim prognosis in the office with Lisa and Mrs. Chandler, and although Mrs. Chandler seemed to have accepted her fate, Lisa had refused to acknowledge that it was not going to be possible to beat this cancer. No matter how Dr. Simmons phrased her message, Lisa hadn't been able to accept that her mother's cancer was past the stage where chemotherapy or radiation would be effective. Further, Mrs. Chandler had always changed the subject when the issue of end-of-life care was raised, passing off the decisions to be made at another time or deferring to Lisa when it came to making any final decisions. When Dr. Roberts himself had tried to broach a discussion of end-of-life care in the hospital, he had met the same barriers.

Dr. Roberts snapped back to the present, looked at his newspaper, and threw it over the side of the bed. He thought about Lisa and Sam. They were still going full speed ahead. Nothing had changed. There was nothing life support could offer her except prolongation of death. It was pretty rare for patients with such severe disease to end up on a vent, but when it happened, it was usually disastrous. Perhaps tomorrow Lisa and Sam would have had more time to comprehend what was happening. He reached over to his bedside lamp, switched it off and flopped himself down on his pillow, waiting for sleep to take him into the next day.

Once Mrs. Chandler was transferred to the ICU, a new resident was assigned to the case, Dr. Hannah Griggs. Mrs. Chandler's problem list grew longer and longer by the hour and Dr. Griggs got each and every page from the nurses. Throughout the first night, the situation grew more and more desperate. Mrs. Chandler's blood pressure dropped significantly, and she required medications, called "pressors," just to maintain a safe blood pressure. Mrs. Chandler was receiving great amounts of fluids and the maximum of three pressor agents simultaneously. Everyone thought for sure Mrs. Chandler was going to die that night.

Lisa and Sam were still vigilant by the bedside, and Dr. Griggs asked them to join her in the family conference room so that she could give them the most recent update. She could tell they were anxious to hear what she had to say, so she wasted no time with pleasantries.

"I wish I had good news for you, but unfortunately things have gone downhill over the course of the night. Right now, your mom requires a lot of medication to keep her blood pressure up and her heart beating. Her lungs have completely failed, and she is one hundred percent dependent on the ventilator. We are doing everything we can to support her, but her body is systematically shutting down. I've also added some broad antibiotics, just in case she is brewing an infection that we aren't yet aware of, but most of her problems are resulting from respiratory failure at this point."

She paused to try and read their reactions. She saw no indication from Lisa or Sam that she shouldn't continue, so she went on.

"I'm doing my best to get her through this, but I want to make sure it's clear to you that I'm not hopeful that she can recover. I'm very concerned that her heart might stop tonight, and if that happens, I would have to perform CPR and possibly give her electric shocks if she has an arrhythmia. If that were to happen, we would compress her chest in order to physically push on her heart to keep it beating, sometimes causing ribs to break. Is this something you would want us to try if it got to that point?"

She held her breath as she waited for the answer, but Lisa and Sam both vigorously nodded their heads.

"All right, that's what we will do then, but I want to make sure you understand that she is dying from her cancer, and I don't feel that those interventions are going to make a difference in her outcome." Dr. Griggs made this last ditch effort to change their minds.

"We understand she is sick right now," Sam finally said, "and we would like all measures to be taken to keep her alive. Her body will fight. God will see to that. Please continue to do everything you can. She is not going to die tonight. The Lord is with her, and we will pray. She'll be just fine."

Once Dr. Roberts arrived the next morning, Dr. Griggs filled him in on the events of the last several hours, including the meeting in the conference room. He went into Mrs. Chandler's room and saw her tiny body amidst the machinery and glanced quickly at the monitor. Her blood pressure was extremely low despite the pressors. Next, he looked at the IV drips to confirm the medications were as Dr. Griggs had reported.

Finally, he forced his eyes over to Mrs. Chandler herself, as devastating as it was to look. She looked even more pathetic than the last time he had seen her, which he hadn't thought possible. She looked like a woman at the end of her line. The ventilator tube jutted out of her mouth, with the strap cinched tightly around her jaw, indenting lines into her face. Her clavicles protruded from her chest wall like two lead pipes. Her eyes, sunken and dark, were only halfway closed, and they looked like glass through the veil of sedatives. Dr. Roberts watched her chest rise and fall to the drum of the ventilator. The alarm on the vent was going off after every second or third breath, and he knew this was a sign that she was uncomfortable. She was "bucking the vent," as we call it. Her body was rejecting the machine's efforts and was trying to fight it, even through the sedatives. Dr. Roberts looked at the settings and made a few adjustments. As he did so, Lisa and Sam entered the room.

"Dr. Roberts!" Lisa exclaimed. "Look what they did to her!"

He didn't know how to respond.

"Ever since they put in that tube, she has been a mess," Sam added.

"This is typically what happens when someone as sick as your mom gets put on life support," Dr. Roberts explained. "It's not a benign process. The body undergoes quite a shock, and we usually try to avoid putting end-stage cancer patients on life support for this very reason."

"But she just needs a few days to rest her lungs and they'll take the tube out, right?" Lisa said.

"Well, that's very unlikely, I'm afraid." Dr. Roberts said.

"We want to try," Lisa interrupted. "She was breathing fine yesterday, and we simply want to get her off the ventilator."

"One step at a time, Lisa. Let's first try to get her settled down on the ventilator. She is fighting against it, and we need to fix the settings to fit her body," Dr. Roberts said. He wasn't about to start the conversation about how medically futile this whole process was already. Clearly, Lisa and Sam wanted to push forward, so he decided to set small goals for them to focus on during what was to be a long process. He explained in detail about what it meant to be "bucking" the vent and that his first priority was to make their mom as comfortable as possible on the machine before even discussing any further plans. Lisa and Sam agreed and thanked him for his efforts to "make her better." He left the room feeling defeated.

After a full week of making little to no headway in weaning Mrs. Chandler off the ventilator, Drs. Roberts and Griggs decided to have another family meeting to discuss the possibility of discontinuing life support and starting Mrs. Chandler on a morphine drip to ease her pain. The fluid surrounding the lung had been removed, and it hadn't made one bit of difference. According to Dr. Simmons, Mrs. Chandler was too sick for them to attempt any further chemotherapy or radiation treatments, and so Dr. Roberts wanted to try and readdress the goals of care.

"You have *obviously* been talking to Dr. Simmons." Lisa was snide at the mention of turning off the machines. "We have no faith in her, you know, and now we have no faith in *you!*"

Dr. Roberts dropped his head. There wasn't much reasoning with Lisa. Every day that he had been seeing Mrs. Chandler, he had been more and more pessimistic with his updates to Lisa and Sam in hopes of convincing them that things were getting nowhere. Their mother simply was not getting better. True, she was alive, but she was hanging on by the thinnest of threads. He hated inflicting suffering, and it felt wrong to continue this woman's life in such an artificial and painful way. Mrs. Chandler's face would grimace with even the slightest touch, which made it impossible even to attempt lifting the sedatives to attempt a weaning trial. He had to get through to them, to explain that there was nothing medicine could do to restore her to the way she was, but neither Lisa nor Sam would believe him. He sincerely hoped that perhaps today they would be able to hear his words.

He had just finished a monologue about feeding tubes. Mrs. Chandler had had no nutrition for over a week, but surgery to place a feeding tube was not a good option for Mrs. Chandler. There is no evidence to support the notion that feeding tubes do anything to prolong the life of patients with end stage cancer. Especially when they are on life support.

"So you want to starve her to death?" Lisa said.

"She can't survive without nutrition," Sam agreed, looking blankly at his mother lying on the bed.

"She can't survive at all," Dr. Roberts answered. Dr. Griggs nodded in agreement.

With that, Lisa erupted in a stream of accusations, each more ludicrous than the next. She was screaming so loudly that the nurses in the next room began to cluster around the room to get a glimpse of the action.

"Why aren't you getting her off the vent?" Lisa began, "Why aren't you increasing her pain medicines? Why aren't you able to get the blood pressure up? Why are you giving her so much fluid? Why are the nurses only washing her once a day?" She fired them off like a machine gun.

Dr. Roberts' face reddened as Lisa grilled him with more and more questions. With each one, he tried his best to answer. But no matter how Dr. Roberts answered Lisa's questions, she was dismissive of his answers and went on to the next accusation.

"I can't talk to you anymore," he yelled back at her, finally. "I've had enough!" He stormed out passed the nurses in the hallway, who stared in shock as he stormed out of the unit in a huff. This was completely uncharacteristic of Dr. Roberts, who was so tolerant and patient with families. Dr. Griggs and the nurses could only stand by and wonder what would happen next.

Dr. Griggs slid out of the room behind Dr. Roberts, whom she had never seen lose his temper before. She couldn't believe what had just happened. Lisa and Sam had already sworn off Dr. Simmons. If they weren't speaking with Dr. Simmons or Dr. Roberts anymore, whom *would* they speak to?

Dr. Roberts sat at his desk with his hands in his head. He was so angry he couldn't concentrate. His confrontation with Lisa and Sam was still ringing in his ears. He looked at the pile of papers in front of him, and he tried to concentrate on being productive, but the conversation with Lisa and Sam wouldn't leave his mind. It was 6:30 at night, and he'd had a long day. His wife was waiting for him, and he longed to just throw on his winter coat and head home for a quiet meal. Instead, he picked up his white coat, put it on and headed back to the intensive care unit.

"I apologize for losing my temper," he said as he walked into the room. "That's not the way I am, and I'm truly sorry. Let's try and start over, from the beginning, because we need to find a common ground so we can help your mom."

Lisa remained silent.

"We're sorry, too," Sam said. "We just don't want to hear that she is going to die and we are not ready to give up on her."

They were the decision makers, and Dr. Roberts knew he had to respect that. But as a doctor, he had to voice his concerns.

"We're not giving up on her; in fact, what I'm suggesting is what I believe will help her," Dr. Roberts said, "and, in fact, my concern is that we are hurting her. De-escalating aggressive measures isn't the same as giving up, Sam. It's important for you to realize that. Giving up would be just walking away. I'm suggesting that we focus our treatment on things that may help relieve her suffering. Putting in a feeding tube, for example, is going to subject her to an unnecessary surgery since she has virtually no chance for an extended survival."

"That's not for you to decide," Sam said respectfully. "That is not for you or me to decide. It's up to God."

Dr. Roberts wouldn't disagree with that.

"We want to give her a chance," Sam said, looking at Lisa. "We want the feeding tube."

"Okay, Sam. If that is what you want, then I'll call the surgeons first thing in the morning," he said, giving up. "Are we okay, now?" He was hopeful that at least the hostility was dwindling.

"Yes, doctor." Sam said. "Thank you very much."

And with that, Dr. Roberts was dismissed.

Ever since I had intubated Mrs. Chandler I had been visiting her daily in the unit and getting updates from Dr. Griggs. I wasn't Mrs. Chandler's resident physician anymore, Dr. Griggs was, but I still felt like Mrs. Chandler was my patient. I would pop down after rounds with Dr. Simmons and visit Mrs. Chandler to see what had become of her.

It was not long after the feeding tube was in place, Dr. Griggs told me that the nurses had called for an ethics consult. As a group, they were so disturbed by the pain and suffering, directly and indirectly inflicted by the life-support systems on Mrs. Chandler. Making matters worse, she had oozing, purulent bedsores. Her limbs were swollen and spongy from the fluid seeping out of her blood vessels and into her tissues and she appeared to be suffering, and the nursing team thought that with each touch, they were contributing to her torment, and so, as a group, they decided to make the call to the ethics committee. A panel of doctors, nurses, clergy, ethicists and hospital administrators would review Mrs. Chandler's case and apply checks and balances to make sure that humane and ethical standards were met.

Dr. Simmons called to let me know what was happening. "The nurses called an ethics consult about Mrs. Chandler," she told me. "They feel like the family isn't acting in the patient's best interest. The nurses say they feel like we are torturing Mrs. Chandler by keeping her alive when everyone knows she's never going to recover. I'm glad they called ethics." Dr. Simmons said.

Dr. Simmons had had a close relationship with Mrs. Chandler long before her patient had become the debilitated woman lying in that hospital bed. I wondered if she regretted not insisting on confronting end-of-life issues with Mrs. Chandler and Lisa in her office before things had gotten to this point, yet I had no doubt that without Dr. Simmons' care and persistence, Mrs. Chandler would not have survived as long as she had. I was glad to hear that Dr. Simmons wasn't offended by the ethics consult and was instead embracing it.

"So, when is it going to be?" I asked.

"I think sometime today. I'll give you a page, if you'd like to come," she offered.

"Oh, definitely. I'll be there," I said. I just hoped nothing happened with any of my patients that would prohibit me from going.

Luckily, nothing came up, and I was able to make it down to the unit when Dr. Simmons paged me later that day. Familiar faces greeted me outside Mrs. Chandler's room. Several of the unit nurses, as well as Dr. Simmons, Dr. Roberts, and Dr. Griggs were all lingering in the nurses' station, waiting for the meeting to commence. Dr. Laramy, the assigned meeting chair, motioned us over to where he was standing at the entrance to the ICU conference room. One by one, we filed in as Dr. Laramy held the door open, as if granting admission. Dr. Simmons and I were the last two to enter when he shut the door, blocking Dr. Simmons' entry.

"Uh, Sara, the family just informed me that they don't want you to come to the meeting," Dr. Laramy said apologetically. "We talked about it as a committee and decided that it's probably best for now if you wait outside. They have a lot of hostility toward you, and I'm not sure how much progress we will be able to make with you in here."

Dr. Simmons raised her eyebrows and tried not to show her shock. I could tell she was at a loss for words. I was rather shocked myself; I had been in several family meetings with angry relatives, but never had they prohibited one of the attending doctors from participating. This was certainly uncharted territory.

"That's fine," Dr. Simmons said, trying to hide her pain. I tried to meet her eyes, but she had already turned to leave. I followed Dr. Laramy into the room.

Lisa and Sam were seated at the conference table with two women on either side of them, apparently more family members. None of them met my eyes as I entered, and I wondered if they had seen Dr. Simmons being turned away.

The conference room was barren except for the rectangular table and its surrounding chairs. A sink and counter lined the back wall, and the floor was covered with white tiling. The room felt more like a kitchen than a conference room, and it probably had been at some point, but for now, it was the largest meeting room we had on the floor. The doctors' white coats blended into the background as they leaned against the wall behind the committee members who were seated. There was a strong sense of "us versus them," with the two sides facing off across the table. The tension was thick, and my adrenaline surged.

Dr. Laramy took his seat at the table, across from Lisa.

"I want to start out by having everyone introduce themselves so we all know everyone present," Dr. Laramy began. "I'll start. I'm Dr. Laramy, a nephrologist and the head of this ethics committee. As you all know, we received a call in hopes that we could help bridge communication between the physicians and the family since some feel that this situation hasn't been going smoothly. Their hope was that having a third-party mediation might help ease the situation. I also want to stress that I do not provide any medical care for your mom and I'm a third party, impartial member. I'm here to lead the meeting and address the concerns of both sides."

I studied Lisa and Sam as Dr. Laramy made his speech. Both were sitting bolt upright, arms folded across their chests. Sam wore no facial expression, while Lisa occasionally smacked her lips together in what seemed like an effort to control her anger. Dr. Laramy, on the other hand, was sitting cross-legged in his chair with his hands wrapped around his knee. He looked casual, which was certainly intentional. He was purposefully giving off body language to try and lighten the air in the room, though it failed miserably.

We then introduced ourselves one by one. The two family members who accompanied Lisa and Sam were Mrs. Chandler's granddaughter and niece. Everyone else was familiar to me.

"Okay, now that we are all acquainted, I'd like to begin by having you tell me exactly what you understand about your mom's condition," Dr. Laramy began.

Lisa sat forward. "We want the breathing tube to come out," she erupted.

Here we go, I thought.

"No, before we talk about the breathing tube, I want to know what you understand about your mom's disease and how we *got* to the breathing tube, just so we can all be on the same page," Dr. Laramy insisted.

Sam touched Lisa's arm to silence her. "Her oxygen levels started to drop because she had some fluid building up around her lungs when she was on the seventeenth floor," Sam said, his voice was shaking. It was the first time I had seen him show any sign of nervousness. It caught me off guard to see him breaking down, as it made me realize how incredibly stressful this situation must be for this unfortunate family. Here they were, with no medical or scientific training, having a meeting about their mother, whose care was completely in the hands of doctors that they simply didn't trust. I felt bad for them, sitting across from this army of white coats. I supposed it must be daunting. As angry as their continuous accusations made me, I also felt a new pity for them.

"She was in a lot of pain," Sam repeated "and so she needed the epidural to try and control the pain while reducing the meds. But as soon as that epidural was placed, she went downhill."

Lisa was rocking back and forth on her chair and nodding her head in agreement.

The conversation went on for a few minutes about Mrs. Chandler's pain issues. Dr. Laramy patiently allowed Lisa and Sam to vent their frustrations, and as I listened, I had to fight the urge to defend myself, Dr. Simmons, and my team on the seventeenth floor. I kept quiet, knowing defensiveness would be counterproductive.

"Okay, I understand what you're saying about all that," Dr. Laramy said after awhile. "Let's talk about *why* she has pain to begin with. Let's talk about the cancer in her bones."

"No, we don't want to talk about cancer," Lisa said curtly. "We want to talk about getting her off the breathing tube."

Sam nodded.

"With all due respect, we really cannot talk about one without talking about the other," Dr. Laramy began. "I understand that it's hard to talk about your mother's terminal disease, but it is central to this meeting and, therefore, I have to insist that we discuss it."

Lisa could see Dr. Laramy's firmness and knew they were not going to win this battle.

"Fine," she said, and she raised her arms up in a bring-it-on gesture. "Let's talk about it. She has cancer. So what?" She placed her hands on her hips.

"Regardless of *why* she ended up on the vent, whether it be her cancer or otherwise, we still have to deal with the fact that she has terminal cancer. I'm going to ask Dr. Roberts to summarize his perspective on where she stands now, medically," Dr. Laramy turned to Dr. Roberts and gave him a quick nod.

"Well, it's not good at all," Dr. Roberts said. "She had effusions, or fluid, building up in her lungs, which we've removed, but it's likely to come back. The problem is that she has an enormous amount of tumor in her lung and we have exhausted all our options for treating it. Dr. Simmons feels that Mrs. Chandler can't survive any more treatments of chemotherapy or radiation. Trying to shrink the tumor isn't an option. On top of the disease in her lungs, she is not maintaining her blood pressure on her own, and she requires medications to keep her blood pressure up. Despite those pressors being at full dose, she is still having periods of low pressure, or hypotension. The hypotension is impacting her kidney function and her urine output is going down. All of these are terrible prognostic signs."

Dr. Roberts paused. I glanced at Lisa, Sam, and the family to see if I could find a glimpse of understanding in their eyes. The granddaughter's face was contorted as she held back tears, but other than her, their faces showed no sign of emotion or comprehension. If they did understand, I thought, they weren't going to admit it.

It was Sam who spoke up first. "We all understand that. But we have hope and faith."

Dr. Laramy turned again to Dr. Roberts. "Can you give us your opinion on what her chances of survival are, Dr. Roberts?"

"Well unfortunately, I believe she has a zero percent chance of surviving off the ventilator," he said quietly, but firmly. I saw Sam look over at Dr. Griggs, who nodded in agreement.

"I don't believe in zero percent," said Sam. "Doctors are not in control, and I have a strong faith that God will help her out of this."

Dr. Laramy leaned forward across the table to articulate his next point. "We aren't here to destroy your faith or hope. I want to make that very, very clear. We are here from a medical perspective, and short of divine intervention, which I mean with the greatest respect, there is little hope that she is going to recover."

Silence filled the room, and Dr. Laramy allowed it to linger for a few moments before moving on.

After what seemed like an eternity, he finally spoke. "Let me change topics for a minute here. What do you think your mom would have wanted in this situation?"

"Mom wanted to live. She said so in the emergency room," Lisa said.

"The doctors came in and asked her if she would want to have shocks and CPR and stuff," Sam said, "and she said yes."

"Did she have a living will, or a document where she maybe wrote down what her wishes would be under these circumstances?" Dr. Laramy asked.

"No, we never made one," Lisa said matter of factly. Sam looked to the ground. I wondered if he was feeling regret that no such documents had been drafted. "She told us her wishes in the emergency room. She wanted to live," Lisa said.

These moments were key: Dr. Laramy was establishing Lisa and Sam's substitutive judgment. In the absence of an advance directive or living will, Dr. Laramy would have to determine whether or not Lisa and Sam were making decisions based on whatever they understood Mrs. Chandler's wishes would have been had she been able to make them herself. This was the bare bones of the meeting, the reason we were all here.

"She said she wanted to be resuscitated while she was in the emergency room?" Dr. Laramy asked in confirmation.

"Yes," Lisa and Sam said in unison.

"All right. That's a start. Now, did she ever discuss with you her wishes regarding long-term life support? Did she ever say she would or would not want to be kept alive on machines for a prolonged period of time?"

"Mom wanted to live! She wanted to keep fighting," Lisa said again.

"Yes, but do you think she would want to live in the state she is now? It's an important distinction, because saying she would want to be resuscitated if she had a hope of returning to a normal or even semi-normal state is quite different than what we are talking about here."

"I never asked her that specifically," Sam admitted.

"What do you *think* she would have wanted, Sam? Do you think that this state is one she would consider a meaningful quality of life?"

"I think my mother would have faith in God and that she would want to continue to fight until He took her," Sam responded. "That's what I think."

Religion in medicine has always been a mystery to me. The majority of my patients are deeply religious, but the way they interpret their religion can vary significantly. I puzzled over Sam's response. To Sam, 'letting God's will prevail' meant using science and medicine to its fullest and if she were to survive, it would be God's work. On the other hand, some patients feel that using science and medicine is working *against* God, and that if a patient is fated to survive, it has nothing to do with what we as doctors can do. Those patients chose to remove the machines and 'let God's will prevail'. I wondered about Sam's interpretation as the conversation continued.

"Lisa, do you agree with what Sam is saying?"

"Definitely," she answered.

"Okay, then. We've established that from the information we have, she would want to continue to be kept alive on life support," Dr. Laramy concluded.

Dr. Roberts raised his eyebrows. Dr. Griggs took in a deep breath, and the other doctors were stoic. They all knew it was over. According to Mrs. Chandler's children, her next of kin and thus her legal decision makers, honoring the patient's wishes meant going full speed ahead. Lisa and Sam didn't move. They hadn't yet realized the battle they had just won.

"So we'll continue to do everything we can to keep her alive," Dr. Laramy said.

Now they got it. Grins from ear to ear stretched across their faces. Lisa grabbed for Sam's hand and they let out a few squeaks of joy. The granddaughter and niece put their arms around them in a congratulatory hug.

"So, where do we go from here, doctor?" Dr. Laramy asked turning to Dr. Roberts.

"The next step, I guess, would be a tracheostomy," Dr. Roberts said. "But we are going to have some trouble there."

"What's a tracheostomy?" Sam asked.

"It's a surgical procedure in which a surgeon will cut a whole in your mom's neck in order to place a more permanent ventilator tube," he began to explain.

"We just said we were going to try to get her off the machine! We don't want her to have a *permanent* ventilator!" Lisa exclaimed.

"If we are going to do everything we can to keep her alive, she needs to have a tracheostomy. First of all, the tube she has now goes down her throat and into her lungs. This puts her at great risk for getting pneumonia. After a few weeks, all patients need to be converted to a tracheostomy. The tracheostomy is a hole in the neck through which we connect the ventilator, and it will hopefully make it easier for us to wean her off, if she ever gets to that point. This way, we can just disconnect the ventilator from the tube in her neck, and reattach it if she doesn't do well. With an oral tube like she has now, she would have to be reintubated if we remove the tube and she doesn't breathe on her own. Its much easier to wean someone if they have a tracheostomy, and much safer," he added.

"So, the tracheostomy will make it easier to wean her off the ventilator?" Sam repeated. He hadn't heard the word "surgery" or "permanent," he heard the word "wean." It was a theme with Lisa and Sam, I realized. They would pick and choose what words they would accept. *Cancer,* no. *Fluid removal,* yes. *Permanent,* no. *Wean,* yes. It was frustrating and I curled my toes under my shoes.

"If she stabilizes enough for us to try and wean her, then yes, it would make it easier," Dr. Roberts said.

"Let's do it, then. Can you do it tonight?" Lisa asked.

"That is what I was trying to explain before," Dr. Roberts said, an edge to his voice, "The problem is that no surgeon would do the procedure on her at this point. She is just too unstable. They would have to bring her down to the operating room, but right now, it's not safe to move her. We wouldn't want her to die in the elevator on the way down."

"So what do you have to do to get her more stable?" Lisa asked.

"Well, for starters, she would have to be off all pressors—"

Lisa interrupted. "She was off them for about an hour yesterday! Why didn't you do it then?!"

"She would have to be off them for longer than just an hour. She would have to be off them completely for at least twenty-four hours before a surgeon would even consider doing the procedure."

"Okay, well, let's start moving the pressors down then. I saw the pump was at 15 today and it was at 20 yesterday, so they can probably bring it down some more," Lisa started, talking a mile a minute. "And her pain medication was being turned up too, I noticed. That one went from 5 to 6, and when it was at 5, her blood pressure was ok, so I think if they turn it back to 5 they might be able to fix her pressure! They just aren't trying hard enough!"

She was playing what I call "the numbers game." To play, all you need is an ill loved one and a feeling of helplessness. You come to the ICU for your daily visit, usually to be greeted by someone who is non-communicative and comatose. You arrive and walk up to the bedside. You might hold your loved one's hand. Then, you examine her face, with a quick kiss to the forehead. After you've said your hellos without any response at all, your eyes can't help but go to the monitor. There isn't much else to look at. By now, you know what a normal heart rate is and a normal blood pressure, and the monitor displays the numbers for you to see. Maybe the blood pressure is a little higher than it was yesterday, and it fills you with hope. Next, you examine the pumps and the IV drips, looking at the numbers on the drip poles. The sedation may have come down a little, and the pressors may have gone up. There may be a new drip running and maybe not. The ventilator has ten to fifteen different numbers on it, and over time, you realize that the number in the upper left is the percent of oxygen your loved one requires. The lower, the better. The doctors have told you that before. So, you can make an assessment based on the numbers you see. And you have an idea of what is going on. Down is good, up is bad. Being a doctor is so simple when you play the numbers game.

I've seen this game played often by my patients' family members and I could tell from Hannah's face that Lisa's 'numbers game' was wearing thin on her nerves. It's quite easy to get frustrated when family members try to micromanage their loved ones care and make requests about how we adjust the drips and ventilators. It's easy to lose your temper if you don't take into account the reason *why* they are watching the numbers. How helpless might *you* feel if your loved one can't move or can't talk to you? How would you feel if *all* you can do is watch their stillness? The only thing that changes is the drips and the monitors, so that is what families cling too. It's human. It's the need to help. It's the need to be there for your family member. Maybe it's guilt. But it almost certainly is love.

"Lisa," Dr. Laramy said kindly, "I think this is part of the reason why the physicians have been getting frustrated. You have to trust that they are trying to do what's best for your mom. Believe it or not, they *do* care. They *want* to help. We are all on the same team. They are going to do everything possible to help your mom, but you have to try and leave the medicine part to the doctors. I think it will help everyone communicate better if we can all establish a little trust and a little faith in each other."

Lisa sat back in her chair looking like a scolded child.

"He's right, Lis," Sam said, "We need to back off and let them do their job. We both do." The words were shocking. Did he truly mean it? If he did, then maybe, just maybe things could get better.

"Okay," Lisa said after a period of time. "I'll cut the attitude. I just don't want to talk about shutting off the machines, anymore."

"That's fine," Dr. Roberts said. "We've established that we are going to continue going full force, but like Dr. Laramy said so eloquently, you have to trust us. We can't help your mom if there is no trust."

Lisa nodded, and for the first time, I saw that she understood and maybe even felt some remorse for being so combative. I could tell by the way her face changed, the way her eyes softened, that she was going to try to trust. My heart flooded with hope.

"We're going to try to wean down the pressors, and once we do, we'll attempt to get the tracheostomy in, okay?" Dr. Roberts said.

"Okay," Lisa said. She smiled broadly and then said "Thank you. Thank you so much."

Three days later, Mrs. Chandler's kidneys shut down, and she was placed on continuous dialysis. A labyrinth of tubes adorned the machine's front panel, one of which was connected to a large catheter placed in Mrs. Chandler's groin. Blood from her femoral vein was sucked out through the catheter and snaked through the tubing into the large, medieval looking contraption. Whizzes, whirls and beeps filled her room as the filter detoxified her blood, doing the job of her failed kidneys.

Mrs. Chandler survived amidst the bags, tubes, machines, and drips that surrounded her. She gaped up at the ceiling, her eyes fixed above her and her jaw hanging open from the pressure of the ventilator tube in her mouth. She now required eight IV drips, a feeding tube, and two machines to keep her body alive. But what about her spirit: Was it still with us, or had it left long ago? What would she say if she could see herself from above? Was this truly what she meant in the emergency room when she told the doctors that she wanted to be resuscitated? There was no way to know, and so her care pressed on.

"I think she is going to go soon. I haven't been able to keep her pressure above sixty systolic, and her body temperature is only ninety-six degrees. I really don't think she is going to make it much longer. I think you should call the family in." The nurse had called Dr. Griggs with the inevitable.

While she was waiting for Lisa and Sam to arrive, Dr. Griggs helped to change the padding underneath Mrs. Chandler's legs. Her skin was so edematous and soggy that fluid was continuously seeping out of her pores. Her legs had blisters that were so fragile, even the most gentle of touches would make them burst. This was a result of her poor nutritional state, even despite the feeding tube. The nurses knew that the sight of the edema upset Lisa and Sam tremendously, so they always made it a priority to change the pads.

When Lisa and Sam arrived, Dr. Griggs was relieved that they'd made it in time. Over the last hour, Mrs. Chandler's blood pressure had been dramatically low, and any minute her heart would stop.

Brother and sister ran to the head of their mother's bed and kissed her head.

"We're here now, Mom. Hang on!" Lisa said.

Sam began praying as he held her hand, the fingers blue from necrosis.

"Her blood pressure has been very low for the last hour or so. The blood isn't getting to her organs, including her brain. The body can't sustain a low blood pressure like this for very long," Dr. Griggs said softly. She quietly left the room amidst their tears and prayers.

Just then, both Lisa and the telemetry monitor began screaming.

"I'm going to have to ask you to step outside now," Dr. Griggs told Lisa and Sam. A nurse had already begun chest compressions. Mrs. Chandler's tiny body was like an elastic band under the force of her compressions.

"Save her!" Lisa yelled, as another nurse pried Lisa and Sam away from the head of the bed.

"They will, Lis, don't worry," Sam assured her.

Once they were out of the room, Dr. Griggs turned to one of the other nurses that had come in to assist in the code.

"Epi, please," she said solemnly.

The nurse nodded and opened the code cart to prepare the drug.

"Epi in," she said quietly.

"Continue compressions," said Dr. Griggs. She could hear Lisa and Sam sobbing directly outside the door. She was very aware of their presence and saw Lisa peeking into the room.

Just then, a loud crack filled the air.

"Someone take over," the nurse gasped, tired from the compressions. "I just broke her rib."

"It happens," Dr. Griggs said, trying to be reassuring. The nurse nodded, but Dr. Griggs could tell she didn't feel any better about the crack she'd heard and felt under her hands.

Codes are usually chaotic and loud. They're often filled with people shouting, needles flying, and IV lines being placed urgently. There's always motion, noise, and commotion. But this scene was just the opposite. There wasn't much to be done. Dialysis had already been running for a week. They had plenty of lines and there was no need for new labs. The drips were all already running and other than chest compressions and the occasional epinephrine or atropine, there wasn't anything to reach for. For eighteen minutes, Dr. Griggs alternated between epinephrine and atropine and ran the code by the book. But the whole time, there was no pulse.

"I'm going to call it, but let me go talk to them first. Keep going," Dr. Griggs said as she left the room.

Lisa and Sam were right outside and had heard everything.

"I'm going to stop the code now," Dr. Griggs said evenly. "She has no pulse and we can't continue this. She has been down for eighteen minutes, and the heart and brain are dead. Only the compressions are moving the blood through her body. I'm really very sorry."

"No, keep going! You haven't been trying long enough. You can't stop now," Sam urged while Lisa screamed through her tears.

"I'm sorry, Sam. But there is nothing I can do. She is gone," Dr. Griggs said firmly.

Lisa darted away from the unit door, and Sam followed her. Dr. Griggs watched as they went, feeling terrible for all that was happening. She returned to the room and instructed the nurses to stop.

The code ended, and everyone stood motionless, looking at Mrs. Chandler. Her struggle was over. One nurse reached over to turn off the dialysis machine and another disconnected the IV drips from the lines. Just then, Sam and Lisa rushed in.

"She's not gone!" Sam said. "God is with her and he will bring her back to us!" He was almost hysterical.

Dr. Griggs knew what she had to do. She reached for the Doppler machine, which is a tiny ultrasound probe that accentuates sound so you can hear the heartbeat. She held it over Mrs. Chandler's carotid artery and turned up the volume. There was nothing but silence.

"Listen," she said softly. "There is no pulse. She has passed away, and I'm really sorry. We're going to step out now and give you some time with her. Take as much time as you need." Dr. Griggs motioned to the nurses, and they left the room, leaving Lisa, Sam and Mrs. Chandler alone.

After a few hours, Dr. Griggs decided it was time to speak with Lisa and Sam. The sobs had softened then vanished completely over the last hour and Dr. Griggs knew she had to ask Lisa and Sam about autopsy. They hadn't yet emerged from the room, but it was nearly 7 a.m., and the paperwork needed to be completed. Legally, every family must be offered the opportunity for an autopsy to be performed on their deceased loved one. Dr. Griggs was certain that Lisa and Sam would want the autopsy. After all the accusations and all the suspicions, it was perhaps the only way they would get the answers they so desperately craved. Dr. Griggs was prepared to do whatever Lisa and Sam wanted her to do. Perhaps the autopsy information would give them some understanding that there was truly nothing more they could have done for their mother. Maybe they needed a report to help them understand the severity of her cancer. She only hoped it would help them move on and recover from their loss. Just one last intervention.

As she entered the room, Lisa and Sam sat by Mrs. Chandler's body, one on each side, holding her hands in unison. The stillness was overwhelming.

"Um, I need to ask you about autopsy," she stuttered.

Lisa looked up from her mother's face and met Hannah's eyes. "No," she said. "She's gone. There's no need. We don't need to make her suffer any more." "Yeah, she has found peace and we don't need to do anything more," Sam agreed. "We've done all we can do. We want to let her rest."

"All right, then. I'll be outside if you need anything." Dr. Griggs was stunned yet heartened by this final decision. She was suddenly overwhelmed by affection for Lisa and Sam that she hadn't realized she ever possessed. She had come to know them, and even though they had asked for the impossible, she felt compassion and some measure of understanding.

"Go ahead and rest, Mom," Lisa told her mother. "You've earned it."

We all have, Dr. Griggs thought, as she headed back to her call room to finally get some rest of her own.

* * *

Even though it was several years ago, Mrs. Chandler's saga and face are still vivid in my mind. Dr. Roberts and I talk about her often as we encounter other patients with situations similar to hers. Mrs. Chandler's story, believe it or not, is not as rare or uncommon as you might think. I've met many "Mrs. Chandlers" through the years, each with a different background and different players in the decision-making process, but all with similar dynamics and similar barriers. Whether they are barriers from the patients themselves or the families who love them, the hospital rooms are riddled with grief, despair, helplessness, and denial.

When we talk about Mrs. Chandler and others like her, Dr. Roberts and I wonder: how and why does it all go so wrong? As we ponder the reasons why people make the choices that they do, our discussions always seem to boil down to the importance of preplanning. The terminal nature of disease is not an easy thing to face, but in order to achieve a peaceful passing, advanced thought and planning is an absolute essential.

Clearly, advance directives and living wills are just one small piece of the overall picture, and too often physicians and patients falsely rely on these documents to set their wishes into action. Discussions between physician and patient are crucial, saving the family endless grief and the necessity of guesswork or even having to defend their decisions, as Sam and Lisa did. Although unpleasant and hard to initiate, these discussions between doctors, patients, and their families serve as the core in preventing situations of uncertainty and desperation as a loved one is dying.

This begs the all-important question: who should initiate these conversations? Is it the doctors? The patient? The families? Certainly, it is the responsibility and obligation of the physician, the patient's primary care physician, the specialty physician, and the hospital physician. The doctors have the experience and the expertise in their daily lives and careers that facilitate meaningful discussion, but too often, the topic of end of life issues gets set aside.

Perhaps the hesitance and relucatance on the part of physicians to initiate these difficult discussions comes from not wanting to give the impression of giving up or admitting defeat to a disease. The feeling of helplessness is hard to reconcile, and as physicians, our instinct and sometimes our training lead us to act in an effort to help. Perhaps these emotions push the initiation of end-of-life discussions to the wayside far too often.

Yet many studies have shown that patients prefer their doctors to bring up the topic of end-of-life care. Meanwhile, it is the role of friends, family, and the patient, too, to be accepting of the topic, not to be fearful of it, and to embrace the concept that none of us are going to live forever. And if the doctor fails in this regard, patients and their families should feel empowered to take the reigns and ask to discuss end-of-life issues. The responsibility is shared, and to wait until it is too late does a disservice to everyone involved. It's hard to imagine that anyone would wish to die under the circumstances that Mrs. Chandler did, and I can't help but wonder if her story may have ended differently had her desires, fears and wishes been shared with her doctors and family. Initiating a candid discussion might be all that is needed to prevent an undignified or painful dying experience.

Understanding the distinction between a patient like Bruce, who had a good chance for survival, and one like Mrs. Chandler, who didn't, is a vital part of any discussion. Considering the long-term outcomes and expectations for recovery is a critical component of medical decision making, one we may push to the back of our minds in the heat of the moment while we are fighting just to maintain the beating heart. As Bruce taught me early on in my training, people can endure tremendous pain and suffering as they inch towards recovery, but even if Mrs. Chandler were to recover, what exactly would her recovery be? Would it be meaningful? Would life be worth living to her? She certainly would never get out of bed again. She would never be pain-free. She would always have widespread cancer. She would most likely never be well enough to leave a hospital or nursing home. Would this be enough for her?

Would it be enough for you or your loved one?

Discussion Questions

1. How did you feel and what emotions did you experience when reading Mrs. Chandler's story?

2. Much of Mrs. Chandler's story could have been different if she and her family were more prepared for the terminal nature of her illness. Why do you suppose there was so much conflict and turmoil surrounding her end-of-life experience? Consider the role of a living will or advanced directive?

3. Lisa and Sam had difficulty recognizing that Mrs. Chandler would not recover from her terminal cancer. What role does hope serve for families facing terminal illness or the impending loss of a loved one?

4. Lisa and Sam's religious faith influenced the medical decisions they made for their mother. Consider and discuss the role of faith in medicine and science.

5. Lisa said that Mrs. Chandler wanted "to live." Think about what "living" and quality of life mean to you. How would you want to be cared for if you were in Mrs. Chandler's situation? What would you want your family to know?

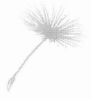

3

A Courageous Choice

Terry braced herself against the shower wall as she held her son. His nineteen-year-old body was small and thin, but she felt unsteady supporting him as the water showered down on them. She hadn't done this in a long time; in fact, she couldn't remember the last time Patrick had asked for help with bathing. But tonight, he needed her arms around him. He wasn't strong enough to stand against the streaming water.

Terry held Patrick tightly, pushing her own body against the wall to prevent them from slipping. The air was steamy, and Patrick was playing feebly with the soap, trying to lather up his arms. His weakness was overwhelming and the medications in his system were making him groggy and confused.

As Terry fought to maintain her balance, Patrick began hacking. The humidity in the shower was loosening the mucus that pooled in his lungs, so she held on tightly in preparation for the next coughing fit. Patrick leaned forward and coughed so fiercely that Terry could feel the pain in her own ribs. Terry closed her eyes to look away. If the mucus was coming, she didn't want to see.

Terry longed to be back on the sofa with Patrick, where they had been just hours before, watching movies and playing cards with his cousins. But instead, she struggled with holding him, praying that she wouldn't drop him as his hacking erupted into a massive fit. When the shaking got to be too much, Terry had to slide down to the ground with him; she simply could not hold Patrick up any longer. Her son sat at her feet, choking in air between his gasps.

And then, like a scene from a scary movie, green nastiness erupted from deep within his lungs. Patrick wretched and shook as Terry looked on in horror. It was endless and unlike anything Terry had ever seen. Having taken care of Patrick and his cystic fibrosis for the past nineteen years, Terry was no stranger to mucus. But *this*, well, this was a whole different ballgame.

For the first time, Terry felt scared. She held Patrick tightly, shocked that so much *junk* could be pooling inside her child's lungs. She closed her eyes and prayed, waiting for the hacking to stop and for Patrick to be calm.

After a surreal eternity, Patrick finally stopped coughing and his breathing slowed to a calmer pace. It was over. Terry felt weak in her knees, but pulled herself together and reached forward to shut off the shower. Patrick remained seated, sobbing in the tub as Terry stepped out to get a towel for him.

While her back was turned, Patrick attempted to pull himself up in the shower. She turned back just in time to see him try and shot her arms out to him just before he slumped into her. She wrapped the towel around him and embraced him, comforting him as she patted him down and held him close. Terry's memories raced back to the day she had brought him home from the hospital for the very first time, wrapped in his baby blanket, cooing as she had patted him, oblivious to the journey that two of them were about to embark upon.

Terry was still a child herself when Patrick's pediatrician, Dr. Cramer, first used the words *cystic fibrosis*. She had delivered Patrick when she was only seventeen years old, and the thought that her baby could possibly be sick had never even crossed her mind. But by the time he was nine months old, Patrick had contracted pneumonia seven times, so it was no surprise to Terry when the doctors wanted to run some tests. Terry had gotten quite an education over the previous nine months, so she knew the drill. When baby Patrick first came crashing into her life, she had no idea how much time she would be spending in doctors' offices, but she was used to it by now.

Dr. Cramer handed her a slip of paper that had the name of a lung doctor scribbled on it, along with a series of lab tests. Dr. Cramer had already told Terry that he wanted to test Patrick for cystic fibrosis, but Terry had just blown it off. Patrick couldn't possibly have such a *bad* condition, she'd thought. Now she froze when she saw the test's name scribbled on the paper Dr. Cramer handed her: "sweat chloride."

Patrick had cystic fibrosis, she was certain of it.

Her mother's voice echoed in her ears. "Hand over my little salty-kins, Terry!" she would say, arms reaching out for her grandson. It was Terry and her mom's nickname for Patrick. He tasted salty when you kissed his soft skin, and the doctor was testing for sweat *chloride*. Terry knew enough chemistry to remember that salt was made of sodium chloride, and the thought throbbed in her mind as she gaped at the words. Now that she knew Patrick had cystic fibrosis, she was afraid to ask the doctor what it *was*.

"Any questions?" Dr. Cramer asked.

Terry shook her head.

"Okay, well, I'll see you back after you've had the tests and met the lung doctor," he said, smiling. He had no idea about "little salty-kins" or what was going on inside Terry's teenage head. Dr. Cramer left the room as Terry stared at her child. Patrick was wiggling in his carrier and reaching for a stuffed shamrock. She handed him the toy and he bee-lined it into his mouth. As mother and son made their way out of the office, Terry knew her life would never be the same.

Terry was in the car driving toward Eastern Memorial Hospital for the trillionth time. She could do this with her eyes closed, she thought, rolling down the window to let the night air blow onto her face. She had to make herself wake up. She was exhausted from her shift at the restaurant and wanted to revitalize herself for Patrick's birthday celebration. He would be six today, and even though he was in the hospital, Terry wanted to make sure it was special. She had bought him a new Lego set last night after work, and she couldn't wait to see his face when he opened it. Patrick was always building things, and when he'd finish one project, he would take it apart and start all over again. He loved puzzles, blocks, and connect-sets, and she thought he was sophisticated enough now to build the rocket ship she'd neatly wrapped and put in the passenger seat.

Terry reflected on the progress Patrick had made in the year since his last birthday. He was old enough now to understand that he wasn't like other kids, that he was sick and needed medicine. But he wasn't quite old enough to be angry or bitter. He knew that his friends didn't have to take pills or inhaler treatments but he wasn't surprised anymore when Terry sat him down for his hour-long nebulizer treatments. He would even sit still and wear the mask without a fight. Well, most of the time. He no longer cried during the chest physical therapy, in which Terry would pound on his back to loosen the mucus that plugged his lungs. But despite his medications, inhalers, and physical therapy, Patrick constantly developed upper respiratory tract infections requiring antibiotics, some of which needed to be taken three or four times per day. But he was at that perfect age, Terry thought, when he was too young to feel any sort of bitterness, but old enough to be cooperative.

As Terry drove, she marvelled at the resilience of her youngest child. She thought about how easy it was for him to keep up with his older brother, who was two years older and healthy. Patrick could run and play like nobody's business, and even his hospitalizations didn't slow him down. She had learned so much in the last six years. Now, she felt like an expert on Patrick's disease. After the shock and confusion of his diagnosis had passed, she'd devoted herself to making sure that life went on, and six years later, she was continuing to do just that. For a disease that had once been such an enigma to her, she realized that she couldn't imagine life without it now. After all, it had come from her, and, therefore, it was a part of her.

Cystic fibrosis is genetic, inherited when two parents each possess a hidden mutant gene that passes silently through generations. If that mutant gene is passed on by both parents to the child, then that child will have the disease, which prevents sodium chloride ions' passage through the tissues of the lung's airways. As a result, mucus becomes dangerously thick, clogging up important glands in the lungs, pancreas, and liver, as well as becomes a source of dangerous infections.

The doctors had taught Terry how to administer chest physical therapy to Patrick, which was a painful process in which she had to thump on his back to help break up the thick mucus plugs in his airways. It was hard to hit her own child so forcefully, but she had to do it, no matter how much they both hated it.

Over the years, Patrick had adjusted well to his frequent hospitalizations. In fact, at six years old, Patrick thought there could be nothing better than being in the hospital. The children's ward was colorful and filled with toys and activities. He had all day to play, except when he had to return to his room to receive his treatments. But the rest of the time, it was a tornado of fun. There were video games, board games, puzzles, movies, art projects, and plenty of other children to play with. Patrick was a social kid, and he loved spending time with the other children whether they were his age or not. His days in the hospital could be spent building models and flying paper airplanes. In between activities, he would eat ice cream and other goodies. Bliss.

Terry turned into the hospital parking lot and after a few rounds of circling, she slipped her Volvo into a spot, grabbed Patrick's birthday package, and headed into the hospital. Once inside, she flashed her visitor's pass from the night before at the security guard, who smiled and waved her through the glass double doors leading into the pediatric ward. Even though Patrick had been admitted only twice this year, the security guards still recognized her as she came in.

She entered the hallway and gave a quick wave to Patrick's nurse from the night before.

"Hi, Theresa," Terry called.

"Hi Terry! He did great today! He let me give him all five treatments!"

"Oh, great! Thank you!" Terry turned the corner to hurry down the corridor to Patrick's room. She was anxious to see him and didn't need to chat this morning. After all, she trusted the nurses and knew that they were taking good care of her baby.

"Mom!" Patrick called as he saw her from inside his room.

"Hiya birthday boy!"

"Dad gave me a toy truck!" Patrick was delighted. Gary was Patrick's stepfather, but he'd helped to raise him since Patrick was two. Patrick's biological father had left before Patrick had even been born, which was just as well for Terry. She had plenty of other things to worry about. Not only did she have Patrick to take care of, but she was also a mom to Gary's two other children, Seth and Kara. Seth was two years older than Patrick, and Kara was about Patrick's age. Terry had to make sure that she paid equal attention to her "sick kid" and her "healthy kids." It was a lot to take on, and there were days when she felt so overwhelmed she could barely breathe. But today wasn't one of them.

"A truck, eh?" Terry planted a quick kiss on Patrick's forehead, then turned to greet her husband.

"Hi, honey," Gary said. They exchanged a quick kiss. "How was work?"

"The same. Good tips today, though." Terry turned toward Patrick, holding his gift behind her back.

"What is it?" Patrick squealed.

"Open it and see. I think you're gonna like it!" she sing-songed.

Patrick was tearing into the paper almost as soon as Terry revealed the package to him. Terry took a step back and reclined into Gary's arms. He gave her a soft squeeze.

"A Lego rocket ship!" Patrick exclaimed, "I wanted this so bad! Seth said I probably can't build it, but I bet I can!"

Terry and Gary spent the next hour by Patrick's side, happy to see him so joyful even though his breathing had worsened in the last few weeks. He had another, infection and his pulmonary function tests had gotten low enough that his doctors felt that he needed IV antibiotics and more aggressive nebulizer treatments. But despite being hospitalized, Patrick was upbeat and energetic; it amazed Terry that he could seem so healthy despite being so sick.

"Well, I'm going to go pick up Seth and Kara from soccer practice now that Mom's here," Gary told Patrick.

"Okay, Dad," Patrick replied, not looking up from the Lego box.

"I'll be home in a few hours," Terry offered. "You can heat up the leftovers from last night for Seth and Kara, okay?"

Gary said he would then gave Patrick a kiss and Terry a wave as he left. Terry and Gary had to tag team often to keep the family running smoothly. Between the two of them, there was always somewhere to be, someone to pick up or some activity to attend.

"Seth and Kara aren't coming?" Patrick asked.

"Not tonight. They're going to come tomorrow after school, but they have to finish their homework once they get home since it's a school night. But we're going to have a big birthday cake when they come tomorrow night, and Grandmom is coming too," Terry answered, hoping that Patrick wasn't too disappointed.

"Okay," he said nonchalantly. Terry was watching his face for any signs of disappointment, and as she studied his face, he suddenly let out a yelp so suddenly that it made her jump. She tensed up for a split second but then relaxed as she realized that Patrick's yell was one of excitement as he had just pulled out the directions for the rocket ship.

"This is awesome!" he exclaimed and then erupted into a coughing fit from his sudden outburst of excitement. He began hacking loud, fitful gasps, and Terry watched as his face turned beat red.

Theresa, the nurse, came rushing in upon hearing his distress, and once she saw Terry's relaxed face and Sean's Legos spilled out over his bed sheets, she immediately understood what had triggered his attack. She smirked and put her stethoscope to his chest.

"Oooh, a wheezy birthday boy! I'll get you a treatment and we'll have you fixed up in no time." She reached for the tubing and facemask at his bed stand while Patrick continued coughing and concentrated hard on controlling his breathing.

"Just a . . . short one . . ." Patrick let out between coughs. "I want to build the . . . the ship!"

"First things first, Patrick. Take your treatment," Terry instructed.

Theresa attached the container of liquid medication to the bottom of the facemask. The mask fit snugly around Patrick's nose and mouth, and she tracked the tubing to the machine that would convert the liquid medication into an aerosolized nebulizer treatment for Patrick to inhale. The medication would quickly help decrease the amount of spasm in his lungs and calm the wheezing. After fifteen minutes or so, Patrick would be back to his regular self. But he flopped back in bed, breathing slowly into the mask with an impatient pout. Terry tossed him a sympathetic look, understanding that Patrick's six-year-old brain was yearning to play with his new toy, but knowing that for now, his Legos would have to wait.

As each year passed, Patrick became more and more resistant to taking his treatments. After school, his brother, the neighborhood kids, and he would dump their backpacks in their respective houses and then meet up in the street for whatever they decided was the game of the day. Baseball, soccer, video games—whatever the game was, it began the instant their feet hit the pavement as they hopped off the bus and lasted until dinnertime. They'd race to their houses to see who would be back to play first, but Patrick would always lose.

"Patrick, take your treatment first!" Terry would yell, hurrying to the hallway to intercept the boys as they dropped off their schoolbags. If she didn't get there soon enough, eight-year-old Patrick would be out the door again before she could blink.

"Awww, Mom! Can't I do it later?"

"*Later* is time for the *next* treatment."

One day, Patrick shouted at his mother and stormed out, leaving Terry speechless in the hallway: "You never let me do anything fun, and I always have to stay in and get treatments and I really don't care if I die. I'm going!"

It was the beginning of a perpetual argument that would last for years to come. It was always Patrick versus Mom, or doctors versus Patrick. As he got older, he had less and less patience for his nebulizers, and Terry began to lose control as Patrick asserted his will. It began with testing. He'd skip the afternoon treatment and test Terry every day after school to see just how far he could go. He tested and tested her, and Terry grew more and more weary. She was, after all, a mother faced with an impossible situation. It was either fight with her child every day with the *hope* that maybe the treatments would prolong Patrick's inevitably shortened life at the expense of him missing out on play—or she could allow him to skip his treatments and just be a kid.

As Patrick grew, Terry struggled with the daily battle. He wouldn't listen to her. He wouldn't listen to his doctors. In fact, he barely paid attention during his visits with his pediatric lung doctor. Instead, he'd fiddle with whatever action figure or toy he'd brought along, breathe into the lung function machine at the doctor's request, and promptly return to his toy. Terry's frustration and fears grew day by day. She'd toss and turn at night, pondering over Patrick's pre-pubescent mind and his deadly chronic disease. She saw more and more how Patrick craved normality: he wanted to be like the other kids, free to play when he wanted, and eat without requiring medicine first. As he got older, the hospitals became less fun and more of a nuisance to him. It was painful for Terry to watch the transformation.

Having a child with a chronic disease is hard enough, and often parents take the brunt of it. Terry had no problem with that. She was an achiever, a fighter. She did what she had to do. She had the support of her husband and her mother, and she had her bond with Patrick. But now, that was beginning to shrivel before her very eyes. They fought more than they talked, and Patrick shouted more than he laughed.

Terry hated her role as the enforcer.

Over time, Patrick and Terry began deal-making. As he wore her down, she'd allow him to skip the after-school treatments as long as he promised to allow her to perform his chest physical therapy before bed and get in three treatments a day, as opposed to the five that were prescribed by his doctors. It wasn't ideal, but Terry had made her decision. She was going to allow Patrick to be a kid, and as long as he maintained a moderate level of compliance with his regimen, she would have to be satisfied. All she wanted was for him to be happy and healthy, and if he couldn't be healthy, she at least wanted him to be happy for whatever time he was with her in this life.

By the time Patrick was twelve, he began managing his own disease, showing an understanding way beyond his years. Terry noticed him paying more attention to his doctors and even asking questions at his visits.

"How come you keep giving me different antibiotics?" Patrick asked Dr. Hammond, his lung doctor, as he prescribed one Patrick hadn't taken before.

His question took Terry aback. She actually had been about to ask Dr. Hammond the same question, and her heart swelled with pride at her son's intelligence.

"Well, if I keep giving you the same antibiotic, then the bacteria in your lungs might get used to it," Dr. Hammond explained. "This way, we're constantly exposing them to new drugs so they won't build up a resistance."

Patrick nodded thoughtfully. He had a concerned look on his face that didn't go unnoticed. Both Terry and Dr. Hammond watched as Patrick prepared his next question.

"What is the cystic fibrosis superbug?" Patrick asked quietly, "I heard someone talking about it last time I was in the hospital. They said it's what kills people with cystic fibrosis. Do I have it?"

Dr. Hammond smiled gently. "No, Patrick. You don't have it. The infection is called *cepacia*. It's a special bacteria that's incredibly resistant to antibiotics, which is why they call it the superbug. And you're right, it's very serious, and we are trying to prevent you from becoming infected with it. Normal people can fight off *cepacia* if they inhale it, but in people with cystic fibrosis, it can be deadly. But you don't have to worry about the right now, okay? Your cultures are showing *pseudomonas* infections mostly, and that's why I keep changing the antibiotics. I don't want the *pseudomonas* to become resistant."

Patrick jerked his head in a quick nod and looked over to Terry. It was clear he wanted to change the subject. It was at that moment that Terry knew Patrick understood how serious his disease was. Although he was just a kid, he was also a kid faced with grown-up problems, and Terry realized just how mature he actually was.

After that doctor's appointment, Terry began treating Patrick like a teenager when it came to his decision-making. She had no doubt that he could handle it. He was smart and responsible, and he knew the cost of his choices. The fighting lessened, and their relationship blossomed with a mutual trust and respect. Gone were the days of arguing. Terry let Patrick skip his afternoon treatments and didn't have to hassle him as much about taking his three daily treatments. They were becoming less like mother and son, and more like friends.

By fourteen years of age, Patrick had moved from building Legos to a taking-things-apart phase. He loved to use his hands and was curious about the way things worked. It wasn't unusual for Terry and Gary to come home from work to find Patrick wrapped up in a tussle of wires, cords, and circuit boards. Remote controlled toys were his new favorites, and after steering (or flying) his latest gadget around the house for a day or so, he would disassemble it and then reassemble it back to fully functioning order. But that wasn't always enough for Patrick. Once he finished mastering all his own toys, he'd move on to his sister's toys, much to her dismay.

Whenever Gary would bring home a new appliance or gadget, Patrick would insist on putting it together all by himself. He would carefully pull out the instruction manual and study the diagrams like an architect over a blueprint. And then, he'd dive right in, head first, to whatever the task at hand. Gary would sit back and supervise Patrick, lending a hand only if Patrick asked for help, which he seldom did. He never needed it. He was bright and extremely good at what he did. If he saw a picture of something, he could build it without ever reading the manual, just by looking at the pictures.

But Gary and Terry soon began to realize that Patrick's skill at understanding pictures and diagrams was a mere adaptation. The truth was that Patrick was fourteen and he could barely read. Physically, Patrick was on par with other kids his age. His disease made him skinnier and more frail than the other kids, but he was more than able to keep up with them. When Terry would watch Patrick run and play with the neighborhood kids, she'd often worry that he just might snap in two, but he never did. Coddling Patrick was not her style, and she had made a conscious effort not to hold him back from all the rough boyhood play.

When it came to reading, Patrick was *way* behind. Terry and Gary soon realized that his lengthy hospital stays were beginning to take a toll on Patrick's schoolwork. He was lagging behind the other kids, although he was adept at covering up his deficits. Only if you really paid attention could you realize Patrick's reading and writing skills were inadequate for his age. After all, since childhood he had been in the hospital at least two to three times a year, and now in his early teens, those numbers were rising to more like five or six times a year, and each hospitalization seemed to get longer than the next.

When he did go to school, he would have to leave class two or three times per day to go to the nurses' office to receive his nebulizer treatments and medications, thereby missing up to an hour of class. He'd also have to leave ten minutes before the lunch period began so that he could swallow the pancreatic enzymes he required to properly digest his lunch. It seemed Patrick was out of class more than he was present, and his grades began to suffer.

Despite all of this, Patrick was one of the most popular kids at school. He was well liked by all his teachers and peers and had an active social life. He had tons of friends and was always surrounded by his best buddies and giggling girls. In fact, Shawna, a pretty fourteen-year-old girl, was coming over quite a bit those days, and it didn't take Terry long to figure out she and Patrick were a couple. So, when Terry made the difficult decision to pull him out of school, it was met with quite a bit of pushback.

"What? Why?" Patrick yelled, exasperated when Terry told him that she had hired a private tutor.

"Honey, I know it's not easy, but I've had a lot of discussions with your teachers, and we all agree that it's just too much for you to keep up with class and be in and out for your treatments. Its just not a good situation for you."

"But what about my friends? What about Shawna?" Tears now welled up in Patrick's eyes.

"What about them?" Terry answered. "They will still be your friends. Shawna will still be able to come over. And we've already arranged with the school that you can participate in all the clubs and after-school activities you'd like."

Patrick was silent as he thought this through, eyes down to the ground. Maybe this wasn't such a terrible thing: no classes, but clubs and sports. Terry could see the gears turning in his young mind.

"Let me think about it," Patrick said.

"All right, we can talk about it again after dinner," Terry answered, but the decision had already been made.

By his mid-teens, Patrick was preoccupied with two things: fixing up cars and Shawna. Shawna and Patrick spent hours together, him upgrading her old car, and her watching him as she proudly passed the tools as he called for them. Terry liked the girl a great deal. Academic and highly organized, she did well in school, which Terry thought was a good influence on Patrick. Shawna walked a straight edge and would scold Patrick if he went out drinking with his older friends. Yep, Terry liked Shawna a *lot*. She even brought her along with them on family vacations.

When Shawna and Patrick were both sixteen, Terry and Gary took all the kids to the Caribbean. Terry, Gary, Kara, Seth, Patrick, and Shawna were one big happy family as they jetted to the Bahamas to escape the bitter cold of Pennsylvania. Patrick forgot to pack his nebulizer, and once they reached the hotel room and Terry realized what he'd done, she felt rage building in the pit of her stomach. How could he forget something like his nebulizer? How could he be so irresponsible? She had trusted him to pack on his own bags, and now she felt completely betrayed. Patrick could see the anger in his mother's eyes.

"Calm down, Mom. Let me talk to you about it, okay?" Patrick said, glancing over at Shawna, who nudged him on, as if she knew what he was about to say.

Terry waited for Patrick to speak.

"I purposely left the nebulizer at home," he began.

"What?!" Terry stared at him hard, dumbfounded by his statement.

"Relax, Mom. We are here for only three days, and I just really wanted this time to myself without any treatments. Just three days to be normal. I brought all my other medications, but I just don't want to miss out on the Bahamas by being cooped up in the room with my nebulizer." He searched Terry's eyes for some kind of response. When she said nothing, he continued.

"Don't be mad. Shawna and I have been talking about my cystic fibrosis a lot, and we've decided that I can't continue to be the 'boy in the bubble.' I want to live while I can. I'm not going to be around much past my twenties. I know that, and so do you. So while I can, I want to enjoy myself. I want to be about living and not only about my disease. I'd rather live to be twenty on *my* terms than to be thirty without experiencing life. I just want to be normal. And while we're here on vacation, I want to be on vacation from my cystic fibrosis, too, okay?" His voice trailed off as he saw the tears begin to pool.

Terry wiped the corner of her eye with her index finger, and the tears broke loose and streamed down her cheeks.

"I'm so proud of you, Patrick," she managed to squeak out while holding back her sobs and also her fears. She embraced him tightly, and as he held her back, she felt his tense body loosen in her arms. It was then that she realized how fearful Patrick must have been to tell her what was weighing on his heart. She clenched her eyes tightly as they embraced, and when she opened them, she saw Shawna standing beside her. The women's eyes locked.

Patrick let go of his mom and turned quickly away to hide his own tears. After rubbing his eyes on his sleeve, he turned back toward them.

"Can we go to the beach now, or what?"

Four days after they returned from vacation, Patrick was back in the hospital. His skin was a dark tan, and he could still smell the salt water in his own hair. He had known it was coming. This one would last more than a week, maybe even a month, he figured. But it was worth it. His vacation had been his freedom, and he didn't care that now his breathing test numbers had decreased to dangerously low levels. He felt okay, a little bit of chest pain from the mucus and coughing, but he wasn't terribly symptomatic.

He reached to his bedside table and pulled out his laptop computer. Seth had brought Patrick ten new movies, all burned onto DVDs so he could play them on his computer. Patrick was thrilled that he now had ten more movies not only to watch, but also to add to his archive. He kept a detailed list of all the movies he owned, alphabetized and by genre. Horror was his favorite. He opened the file from his computer and as he finished entering the last of the new titles, Terry popped in for her after work visit.

"Hiya, kid." She plopped herself down on a chair by Patrick's bedside.

Patrick took a look at his mother. Her blonde hair was pulled back in a messy ponytail, and her eyes were heavy from fatigue. She'd been working late nights to complete her college coursework during the mornings. He loved having her visit, and she never missed a day, but he always felt a twinge of guilt when he saw how exhausted she was by the time she arrived. The drive wasn't on her way home from work, and she often had to rush to the hospital and then home to take care of his brother and sister. He knew it was a lot for her, and he felt particularly bad because this hospitalization was, in a way, his own fault.

"Hey, Ma," he answered. "You look beat."

"Yeah. It's been a long day. Did Dr. Hammond come by?"

"Uh, huh," he nodded, "More of the same. IV antibiotics and more nebulizers. Its *pseudomonas* again."

Patrick could see Terry's relief when he told her that the bacteria in his lungs weren't *cepacia*. It was unspoken between the two of them, but they both feared that at any time Dr. Hammond might come in and reveal that Patrick's sputum sample was growing the superbug. The incurable.

"Okay. Well, hopefully it won't be too long this time." She tried to be nonchalant but couldn't hide her relief from Patrick.

They sat silent for a few minutes. The silence was uncomfortable as Patrick wondered if now would be a good time to ask.

"Mom?" Patrick's voice was soft.

"Yes?"

"I've been thinking a lot about my future. Its just a matter of time before I get really bad, and, well, I was thinking I'd like to get married." He was choking out the words and braced himself for Terry's reaction.

"Married?" Terry held her voice steady. She felt dizzy.

"Yeah. We both know I'd be really lucky to reach twenty-five, and, well, I just don't want to miss out. I really want to propose to Shawna. I want to buy her a ring. I want to know what it feels like to propose and to get married. I saved up my money, but I wanted to make sure you wouldn't be mad first."

Terry thought about it. He had a point: true, they were just kids, but even if Patrick survived to be eighteen, the legal age for marriage, he might not be healthy enough to get himself down the aisle.

"Are you sure?" she asked.

He nodded.

"Well, if that's what you want to do, then I'm not going to stand in your way. You should talk to Shawna's parents too, though," Terry answered. She felt like screaming as the words came out of her mouth. This wasn't the way it was supposed to be. Her son was supposed to be a healthy sixteen-year-old boy, not worrying about whether or not he would live long enough to get married. He was supposed to be out drinking beer and getting into trouble. He wasn't supposed to be sitting next to her in a hospital bed asking for her permission to propose to his sixteen-year-old girlfriend.

But life was as it was, and Terry stopped herself from thinking about what should be. Why give herself that kind of pain? Instead, she had to fill her heart with love for Patrick and her other children. So the answer was, of course, yes.

Patrick was seventeen when Shawna broke up with him. She had worn his diamond ring for a year, but eventually, the relationship had fallen apart. Being in the hospital every day with her fiancé wasn't the way she wanted to spend her teen years, and Patrick had even missed the prom because he'd been hospitalized. Eventually, she broke the news to him, and Terry was proud of the way Patrick handled it. He wasn't angry or even bitter. Even though he was hurt, he understood. It wasn't exactly a hard concept to grasp. Patrick was in the hospital more than he was out, and Shawna had an active social life at school. Patrick, on the other hand, was being privately tutored. It just wasn't going to work.

But Patrick was resilient, and it wasn't long before he was out and about again with his brother and friends. There were parties every weekend and whenever Patrick could make one, he'd be there. He wasn't holding back on life by any means.

Sometime after his eighteenth birthday, I met Patrick on the last day of one his longer hospitalizations. Patrick was old enough that he was no longer a patient in the children's hospital. Instead, he was now an adult and wasn't being treated by pediatricians. Gone were the video games and ice cream. Gone were the colorful walls and pediatric nurses. The adult hospital was a much more dismal place than what Patrick was used to.

Walking to his room, I was excited to meet him. As a second-year resident, knowing I wanted to go into pulmonary and critical care, I was eager to begin learning about patients with cystic fibrosis. He would also be a nice change of pace from the all my elderly patients. Since I was in my twenties, Patrick was closer to my age than any of my other patients, and the idea of working with someone so young was exciting to me. Before opening the door, I thought about what kind of conversation I'd try to whip up to build rapport with my new, young patient.

His room was farthest from the nurses' station since Patrick was so young, able to walk on his own and take care of himself for the most part. An isolation cart stood outside his doorway to minimize the chance of infection, and the red sign on his door shouted at me as I gowned up: "CONTACT ISOLATION! Gloves and gowns are required at all times." All routine and expected. I dressed in the familiar yellow garb and knocked on the door.

"Yeah?"

Taking that as an invitation, I opened the door and went in to greet Patrick. The room was dark, and his bed was on the far side of the room. The desolation hit me like a brick. The shades were drawn despite the fact that it was early afternoon. Patrick had his computer on his lap, though, which explained why the room was so dark; he was watching a movie. Screams and blaring music emanated from his computer speakers. I waited for him to turn it down so that I could say hello, but he didn't move.

So I raised my voice over the din. "Hi, Mr. O'Connor!" As soon as I said it, I felt silly. I always called my patients "Mr." or "Mrs.," as the majority of them were vastly older than I was. But Patrick was a teenager, and my gaffe was awkward.

"Uh, I'm Dr. Van Scoy," I stuttered, expecting him to pause his movie or at least look up at me. But he did no such thing. His gaze never left his computer screen.

"How are you doing?" I asked, feeling uncomfortable and annoyed that he wasn't paying any attention to me at all.

"The same." Terse. Flat.

"Are you having any shortness of breath?" I felt stupid and wanted to leave.

Patrick shook his head no.

"Uh, okay, good. Any pain?"

The same head shake.

Okay, what now? "Can I listen to your lungs?"

He leaned forward, exposing his back.

He was wearing a green T-shirt and a pair of sweatpants. Normally, I would place my stethoscope underneath the shirt to get the best listen to the lungs that I could, but in my discomfort, I just placed the bell of my stethoscope on his back.

"Deep breath," I instructed.

He obliged, movie blaring, never looking away from the screen.

I listened to the crackles of mucus as he inhaled and exhaled and looked around his room. A remote-control helicopter and a pile of DVDs sat on the windowsill. Clothing was strewn about, along with car magazines and a portable video game player. None of my other patients' rooms had so much *stuff*.

Patrick leaned back, ending my pulmonary exam for me.

"Uh, all right. I guess I'll come back later." I turned to go.

"Am I going home tomorrow?" Patrick asked abruptly, his eyes suddenly locked on mine.

His sudden interest in me was startling, but I managed. "That's what I hear. I need to confirm with Dr. Hammond, and I'll get your paperwork started."

"Okay," he said, and turned back to the movie.

A screeching damsel in distress bid me goodbye as I exited the room.

After the door closed and I'd stripped off the isolation gear, I stood still for a moment to reflect on what had just happened. I hadn't interviewed him, and I hadn't even really examined him. *What* would I say on rounds? Should I go back in and demand that he allow me to do my job? Could I face Dr. Hammond, my attending? How would I present this patient to him? I had essentially no information about the state of his symptoms or even a decent physical exam!

Perhaps I'd stop back before rounds and see if his movie was over, I decided. In the meantime, I made my way to his chart. When I found it, I had to lift it with two hands because it was so thick. I flipped it open, and papers spilled out from inside the binder. I looked at the admission date on one that came loose: Patrick had been in the hospital for five weeks. *Five weeks.* I turned to the beginning and began to read it all.

Patrick had been non-compliant with his medications for a week before his admission (while he had been on vacation), and his breathing test results had been terrible when he had first been admitted. I'd never seen numbers so low. He'd grown huge quantities of bacteria in his sputum and been on five different antibiotics in as many weeks. He had required a lot of IV medication to control the chest pains he experienced with every breath. As I read through the pages, I saw his daily breathing tests, his daily blood draws, and his vital signs, which had been taken every six to eight hours—all for five weeks. There were many days the nurses documented "patient refused" in the area where his blood pressure and temperature should have been.

As I read, I began to understand the young man in the dark room. A resident had checked on him every day, asked him the same questions over and over, done the same physical exam and told him the same thing: "We'll send you home as soon as your numbers improve." I was just another resident to him, with the same questions and the same answers.

The breathing test result from that day was 50 percent, which was still very low, but acceptable for us to release him from all the tedium of our care. I immediately began the discharge paperwork, knowing that after rounds, Dr. Hammond would give me the green light to send Patrick home.

It took only three weeks after Patrick's discharge for him to find himself back in Dr. Hammond's office. He'd spiked a fever a week before, and Dr. Hammond had requested a sputum sample and that they see him in seven days.

When they were seated, Patrick saw the results of his breathing test on the table: 20 percent. He knew what that meant without being told: he was going back to the hospital. A group of guys were going camping that weekend and he would have to miss it yet again.

When Dr. Hammond came in, Patrick inferred even worse news by the look on his face.

"I have *cepacia*, don't I?"

"Yes, you do," Dr. Hammond confirmed. His eyes were now on the breathing test.

"I'm not going in," Patrick said. "I'm done. I want to be done. I want to go on hospice."

Terry felt her stomach flip and a lump rise in her throat, and she swallowed hard to alleviate the pain. *Hospice* hit her like a Mack truck. To her, hospice meant the place where old people go to die, and now her little boy was saying he *wanted* it, straight out, right in front of her.

Dr. Hammond showed no signs of surprise. "Well, that's an option we can certainly discuss." Cautiously, he looked over at Terry to try and read how she was feeling. She was staring blankly but nodded her head for him to continue.

"Hospice can be a wonderful thing, and if it's right for you, then we'll help get you set up. But first I want to make sure you understand exactly what it means."

Patrick sat up, listening intently as the doctor explained the process, how patients can enter hospice when they have a terminal disease and have a life expectancy of less than six months, how he would be forgoing any attempts at aggressive treatments for his cystic fibrosis and for his bacterial infections, and instead his treatment would focus more on pain and symptom relief.

He listened as Dr. Hammond explained the different settings at which hospice care can occur: home hospice, nursing home hospice, and inpatient hospice. The hospice provider could deliver everything he needed directly to his home and help train his mother how to administer prescribed medications based on his symptoms and pain levels. They would send a nurse out day or night if needed to supplement the regularly scheduled visits. They would even deliver a hospital bed and other medical equipment to his house if they wanted or needed it. Or, if it was too difficult to handle at home, he could go to an inpatient unit.

It sounded like heaven to Patrick. He would need to take medications only to keep him comfortable and wouldn't have to go through all the different nebulizer treatments unless he absolutely needed them and *chose* to take them. This meant that he, not his disease, would have control.

Wanting to be sure he fully understood, he probed, "So, exactly how many nebulizers will I *have* to take?"

Dr. Hammond answered as best as he could, knowing that Patrick's real question was "Just how *normal* can I be?"

After leaving the doctor's office, Terry never questioned Patrick's decision. He was legally an adult and wise beyond his years. Although she had to fight her urge to beg him to try and save himself, to fight longer, she knew how resolute her son could be, and she knew, above all, that spending his remaining time in the hospital was not an option Patrick would entertain. Dr. Hammond felt it was an appropriate and reasonable decision, and Terry felt reassured by her discussions with him. She wasn't a terrible mother for allowing Patrick to forego aggressive treatment, he insisted. And so it didn't take long for Terry to be at peace with Patrick's decision, and they talked about it often and in depth. She was certain he was making the right choice for himself and, as always, offered her unwavering support.

After one of their many conversations on the living room sofa, Patrick turned to Terry with a sparkle in his eye.

"Let's have a party! It'll be a celebration-of-life party. I want to do something really fun. We can rent out the Irish Pub and invite everyone and just have a party." He got more excited as he spoke. "Whaddya think?"

"Sure, Patrick." For a moment, she'd been taken aback, but now she was getting in the spirit. "I think that's a great idea. We Irish can get through anything with a party and a little beer!" She laughed. "Let's do it!"

The hall was booked for three weekends from then, and Patrick invited all his friends and family. The preparations were like a whirlwind; although Patrick was relatively well right now, he officially on home hospice and they both knew that the *cepacia* in his lungs could rear its ugly head at any time. Even though Patrick's "stats" were declining dramatically, his spirit was doing no such thing. Perhaps he couldn't run about, and certainly he had periods of chest pain and shortness of breath, but in the weeks leading up to his big party, he lived pretty normally thanks to the care from his hospice team. The family spent a lot of time together, and Patrick spent almost every night playing cards with his brother, sister, and cousins. Everyone wanted to be near Patrick, and he loved every minute of it.

On the day of the party, the hall was decked out in explosions of green and white. Shamrocks lined the walls, and Irish music blared from the speakers above. Patrick's cousins surprised him by with an enormous banner that read "Celebration of Life" in enormous green, white, and silver lettering. In the spaces between the letters, each family member and friend had scrawled messages to Patrick. It hung boldly on the wall and served as a visual reminder to Patrick of how loved he truly was. As the guests arrived, Terry watched them stand awkwardly, not sure how to act or what to say. Was this a death party? Should they express their condolences to Patrick and his family? What should they say to Patrick? But the instant Patrick greeted them, all those worries melted away.

During the party, Terry watched Patrick laugh and joke with his friends. He greeted each guest as they came to his bash, pointing them in the direction of the food and drink. He was the host with the most, and

Terry and Gary couldn't help but feel pride and love flow through them like a river. The party raged for hours, and by the end of the evening any uneasy feelings of awkwardness had dissolved into fun and laughter. By two in the morning, when Terry could no longer beat back her fatigue, she watched from a table as Patrick escorted the last guest to the door. Terry chuckled to herself as she realized the irony that Patrick was, in fact, the last one standing.

Even though the doctors had prepared them for a rapid and steady decline, Patrick remained stable for the next several months. He took it easy at home, resting often, and he had variable periods of pain and shortness of breath, but it took the doctors by surprise at just how long Patrick remained relatively healthy. Terry called upon the hospice agency only every few days in the beginning, and they'd respond promptly by helping with Patrick's supplies and painkiller dosages. Eventually, though, they were unable to control Patrick's unrelenting chest pain. His cough worsened, which only made the pain worse, and he wasn't able to generate enough force to cough out the mucus in his airways.

It soon became clear that Patrick would require IV pain medications, and the hospice nurse questioned Patrick about how he wanted to move forward. Patrick and Terry both agreed that in order for Patrick to have rest and calm, home wasn't the place to be any more. They had two large dogs running around, and the house was always bustling with activity. Besides, Patrick didn't want to interrupt Seth and Kara's busy lives with hospital beds and IV poles. He was adamant that he wanted life to go on and that he wanted no part of disrupting the natural flow.

Terry was astounded at the ease with which Patrick took to the inpatient hospice facility. When he arrived, he showed no signs of fear or even hesitation. His movements were slow from the pain medications, but he refused to ask Terry or Gary for any assistance getting inside.

They were greeted by the registrar, Karen, as they entered a room off the main lobby. "Hello. You must be Patrick. Dr. Hammond called and told me to expect you. I have your paperwork already and so we can get you up to your room. I know you had a long trip."

She motioned them into a sitting room that looked like it was straight out of a Martha Stewart magazine. Patrick took a seat on the sofa and Terry realized as she watched him collapse into the cushions just how much energy he was expending just to stand and walk.

Karen could also sense Patrick's fatigue, so she dove right into her speech as she handed him a glossy brochure about the facility. "Once you get settled in your room, we can go over this in more detail. If you're feeling up to it, I can give you a tour, and this pamphlet goes into our history and all the amenities, but you can glance through that at your leisure if you're interested. We try to make this place feel like a second home, not only for you, but also for your family. We have a kitchen, a TV room and a small library that you and your family are free to use. Again, you can flip through the brochure upstairs in your room. For now, let's just get you registered.

"Your home nurse sent me over all your home hospice information, so I have copies of all your medical information and insurance information." She was gentle as she spoke, and Terry could see Karen was proceeding cautiously, so as not to rush Patrick or overwhelm him when she handed him some more documents.

After the orientation process was over, Karen led them up to the main wing where Patrick would be staying. The inside of the building was warm and airy, with indoor gardens and large windows. It was clear that they made an effort to make the facility as aesthetically pleasing as possible, despite the reality that the patients here were dying.

As they approached the patient areas, the interior looked more like a hospital unit with nurses, monitors, and nursing stations. There were the usual supplies, IV bags, and medications, but a striking difference was the profound lack of noise. As they walked, Terry could hear Patrick's breathing louder than anything else. Passing the patient rooms, Terry couldn't help but peer inside and feel uncomfortable. All the other patients seemed two hundred years older than Patrick, with heads covered in gray hair and wrinkled skin stained by decades of life.

Terry shuddered as she looked at Patrick and tried to imagine him lying among these old people. Perhaps they had made the wrong decision. Patrick didn't belong here. He was walking, talking. He was the antithesis of what lay in the beds here. He was youth. But he was also dying, and Terry had to remind herself of that as they finally reached his room.

They were greeted by a nurse, Stan, who offered Patrick a hospital gown, which he waved off politely. "No, thanks," Patrick said. "I have my own clothes."

Terry chuckled and smiled at Stan. "Patrick's never worn a hospital gown in his entire life. He's more of a T-shirt and sweatpants kind of kid."

Stan raised his eyebrows. "Well, then!" He smiled and dramatically tossed the gown across the room. "How about *that*?"

For the next few days, Patrick had a constant flow of visitors. In between his shots of morphine, he had friends, cousin, aunts, uncles, and grandparents all coming to visit him in the hospice facility. It got to be so overwhelming that Terry had to limit visitors to immediate family. She wanted Patrick to get to rest, and for the first few days, he spent his entire day with visitors streaming in and out. As the days passed, the hospice nurses increased his morphine as necessary. When Patrick's pain wasn't controlled, he was less interactive and was still, sometimes withdrawn. But as the morphine took effect, Terry noticed a definite improvement in his mental state, and he was able to enjoy card games and movies. He was less breathless with his pain medicine and was able to keep up with the conversations and socialize more than when the drug effects were beginning to abate. The nurses were very much attuned to Patrick's needs and were diligent with administering the medications at just the right time.

During the daytime, Patrick would roam the halls and raid the kitchen for ice cream. Having a patient moving about was quite different for the nurses. Most of their patients were confused, elderly people who hadn't walked in years. But Patrick was a burst of motion, almost a blur as he strolled the hallways of an otherwise motionless ward. By the evening, his energy would dissipate, so he'd spend most of his time on the sofa in the TV room playing games or watching movies with his brother, sister, or cousins.

Terry stayed in Patrick's room every night. The nurses had rolled in an extra bed for her to spend the nights while Gary took the kids home to get ready for school the next day. The dark nights were peaceful for the two of them, and Terry and Patrick could spend hours talking if Patrick had the energy. There were many times that Patrick was still lucid through the drugs, and it allowed for precious conversation that Terry cherished.

At the end of one night's conversation, he asked his mom to help him take a shower, a request that startled her. Patrick wasn't one to ask for help, but Terry was always there to provide him with it, should he need it.

Her son's life was coming to an end, and Terry knew it as she held him there, patting him dry after his shower. The spewing of mucus was over, but there was undoubtedly more to come. He was weaker tonight than she had ever seen him, but the peace he had reached in the last several weeks at the hospice facility and with his family steadied her fear.

She helped him into his pajamas, and he fell asleep as soon as his head hit the pillow, while Terry lay awake listening to his labored breathing. A few hours went by and then Patrick stirred, woke up and in a state of brief confusion, and tried to get out of bed.

"What do you need, Patrick?" Terry sat up on her cot.

"I want some ice cream," he answered, so groggy that his voice seemed unfamiliar.

"Okay, I'll go get you some, but you stay in bed, all right? I'll bring it to you." Terry glanced at the clock: three in the morning. Patrick often craved ice cream in the middle of the night; it was a habit he had picked up from all the years of being at the children's hospital.

When Terry returned from the kitchen with Patrick's treat, she sat on the edge of his bed and gently shook him to wake him. He didn't move. She immediately put her head on his chest to see if he was breathing, and he was. She could hear the crackles of mucus deep inside his lungs. She shook him more vigorously, calling to him, but there was no response.

She jetted to the nurses station and found Lisa, his evening nurse, reading a magazine.

"Patrick isn't waking up!" Terry said, trying to keep her voice from sounding frantic. She had to stay even-keeled; she couldn't panic. She had to accept that Patrick might not wake up, and that Lisa was not able to do anything to reverse it. It was Patrick's wish. It was Patrick's wish. She repeated the words over and over silently in her mind.

Lisa stood up smoothly and headed toward the room. Her calm demeanor was a stark contrast to the chaos in Terry's head, so Terry tried to latch on to Lisa's state of mind and followed her back to the room.

Lisa called out to Patrick, but he did not respond. Her voice was quiet and gentle, and her movements were slow and steady. She placed her stethoscope on his chest and listened. Lisa placed a thermometer under Patrick's tongue and waited until the number flashed on the screen: 104 degrees

"Call the doctor," Lisa directed to the nurse standing at the doorway, "and can you bring in some Tylenol?" The other nurse nodded as she headed to the nurses' station.

"He's in a coma, isn't he?" Terry asked Lisa.

Lisa gave Terry a gentle, direct look. "I can't say for sure yet, but his fever is really high, and that can make him lethargic like this."

Terry clutched her hands together with her eyes riveted on Patrick, hoping he would speak to her. But there was nothing.

"We can put some oxygen on him and see if it helps, if you like. But I know that Patrick hated having to wear the mask."

"Yeah. No oxygen. He hated it. He absolutely hated it," Terry replied. Saying this was difficult. She reached for her cell phone to make the calls. Patrick was slipping away.

The hospice doctor, Dr. Tanner, arrived about thirty minutes later. Patrick still hadn't opened his eyes or stirred. He remained still and peaceful, still wearing his favorite Guinness sweatpants with the shamrock on the thigh. The only noise was a soft gurgling coming from inside his chest.

"Hello, Mrs. O'Connor." He reached out his hand to Terry.

She took and responded quietly. "Hi."

"The nursing team has filled me in on everything that's happened, and it seems that he has a pretty high fever, which may be part of the reason why he isn't responding to us. It could also be that his oxygen levels have dropped."

"Is he in a coma?" Terry was afraid to hear the answer.

"Well, that's a hard term to define, but I'd say he is non-responsive," Dr. Tanner said.

"But what does that mean? Is he ever going to speak to me again?" Terry was surprised at how hostile her words sounded as they came out.

"I wish I could say for sure," Dr. Tanner answered, "but right now I think it could go either way."

It was a non-answer. Patrick had always hated when doctors did this. Just as Terry was ready to ask her next question, Gary, Seth and Kara came rushing into the room. Their eyes were red and the three of them looked dishevelled. As they rushed to his side, the family wept at Patrick's bedside, but after ten minutes or so, the tears subsided and they were left with just them and Patrick, still and restful.

"This was his choice," Gary reassured Terry. "This was the way he wanted it. We shouldn't be making a fuss over him. That's not what he wanted. Let's try and keep ourselves together." He looked over to Kara and Seth and they nodded in agreement.

Within a few minutes, the family was sitting around Patrick's bedside, and on the side of his bed, having normal conversation and talking about Patrick's antics. It wasn't long before the conversation was jovial and they were laughing and joking. Although the nurses had been coming in and out to check on Patrick and his family, it wasn't until a few hours before Lisa approached Terry with a serious look on her face.

This is bad, whatever it is, Terry thought. For a panic-stricken moment her eyes darted to Patrick. Had he died while they were chatting? Was that what Lisa was about to tell her? She heaved a sigh of relief when she saw his chest wall moving rhythmically up and down. Terry turned her head back to Lisa and waited for her to begin.

"Um, Mrs. O'Connor," Lisa began. "I'm going to have to put Patrick into a hospital gown. You see, he's going to need a urinary catheter and it's going to be much easier for us to wash and clean him if he isn't in his clothing . . ." Her voice trailed off.

Terry was confused. That's all? That was it?

"I know how much Patrick didn't like hospital gowns, but—"

Terry cut her off. "It's okay, Lisa," Terry smiled. "He'll understand. He won't like the catheter, but I know he needs it. He can't urinate on his own, right?"

"Exactly. His bladder will get distended and that would be pretty uncomfortable for him," Lisa said.

"All right, but can you do it after the kids leave?"

"Sure," Lisa agreed. "That's not a problem at all."

Terry watched as Lisa left the room. She was touched by Lisa's consideration. Lisa was completely aware of what Patrick would have wanted, and it was clear that Lisa didn't want to do anything at all that would have made Patrick feel pain or be uncomfortable. It was just a piece of cloth, but Lisa took it seriously. Terry knew they had come to the right place. Even the staff understood Patrick. She turned to him and saw him lying there and felt his peace emanating throughout the room.

Patrick had been in a coma for fourteen hours when Seth, Kara and Gary began to pack up their things to return home. Only Terry had been staying nights. Patrick hadn't wanted anyone else to stay. He wanted life to go on and for Seth and Kara to continue to "do their thing," as Patrick would say. Terry walked the rest of her family down to the main exit and hugged them all goodnight. Gary held her more tightly than usual as they said goodbye, and she smiled and waved as they headed to the car.

When she returned back upstairs, she was shocked at what she saw. Lisa had put Patrick in the hospital gown and placed his folded clothing on the table next to him. Now he looked sick, shockingly frail and delicate. With his white skin and dark hair, he looked like a vampire straight out of his own video archive. Realizing that this was the first time that Patrick had looked like someone who was about to die, Terry gathered her composure, checked her fear at the door, and climbed into bed next to her son. His skin was burning up, and sweat was pouring off his body. His body was in crisis.

Throughout the night, Terry spoke softly in Patrick's ear.

"It's all right. You can go. I'll be all right. Things won't fall apart. *I* won't fall apart. I'll take care of everyone. You don't have to worry. We are all going to be just fine."

Patrick died early the next morning. Terry was by his side, holding his burning hand. Exactly when his breathing slowed to a halt and his heart stopped beating was hard to say. The passage from life to death was smooth and quiet; there were no monitors beeping or frantic cries. It was not an event but a transition, Patrick's final transition, and it was perfect in every way.

* * *

Though I met Patrick that day in the hospital, I didn't meet Terry until about two years after his death, when I asked her if I could write about him. As I drove to her office, where she now serves as a social worker, I was filled with anxiety about how the interview would go. How could I ask a mother to tell me the intimate details of her son's death? Would I be able to get the words out to ask my questions? Would she be crying throughout my interview? What would I say to her and how would I console her? What kind of a burden would my interview place upon her? I was filled with uncertainty when I arrived and had to steady my own knees as I shook her hand in greeting.

Yet Terry made me feel comfortable immediately. She related her son's story with what seemed to be remarkable ease. I didn't have to ask a lot of questions, as she was happy to share. I was shocked at how different her demeanor was from the hysterical, grieving mother I'd expected.

When I told her as much, Terry confided that after Patrick died, she'd been surprised by her own reaction. In the weeks and months after he was buried, she'd wondered why it wasn't harder for her: *What's wrong with me? Why am I not grieving more for the loss of my son? Why am I not hugging his pillow at night and smelling his old clothes like the other mothers who have lost children? How is it that I am genuinely okay?*

Terry then answered her own questions for me. She told me about how the process of Patrick's hospice stay had enabled her and her family to accept and embrace his impending death. She was able to ask him questions: Are you scared? What does it feel like? She was able to talk to him and to tell him all the things a mother needs to tell a son. They were able to talk about life and death and to be prepared for what lies ahead. Patrick gave her strength by telling her the way he saw his life.

"I might not have been here long, but I lived life as if I'm one hundred years old," he had told her the night before he died.

Hospice provided Terry with acceptance before the death actually happened. It allowed her time to emotionally and intellectually grasp that he was going to die. It enabled Terry and her family to let go. They had months of closure, months of time to learn to accept the inevitable. Terry told me that all that needed to be said between her family and Patrick had been said. It was the very reason she sat before me answering my probing questions candidly and without hesitation. It was why she maintained her full composure while detailing the way in which her son met death and how she went on afterward.

"People can survive things they can't even imagine," she insisted. "You have no idea what you can endure and stride through until you actually go through it. You see so many movies [about death], but it was nothing like that. It was better than that."

Patrick donated all his organs to cystic fibrosis research. "Let them take it all!" he said, with the certainty that makes his story remarkable. Patrick knew where to draw his line in the sand and knew what he was and was not willing to endure. For Patrick, the idea of lying in a hospital bed maintained by machinery was not one he would entertain. His ability to perceive the world around him and interact with it beyond a hospital setting was what he defined as a meaningful quality of life which guided his choices. Patrick left the world gracefully leaving his family with peace and certainty. His story is a lesson to all of us, illustrating that taking control of one's own medical decisions and planning ahead, whether young or old, can not only relieve your own suffering, but that of your loved ones.

Discussion Questions

1. Patrick knew where his "line in the sand" was and courageously faced it—where is your line in the sand? Why is it important to communicate your wishes to your family and how might you go about doing so?

2. Were you surprised to hear Patrick ask his physician about hospice? What was your initial reaction about Patrick enrolling on hospice? Was his experience what you expected? Would you feel comfortable discussing hospice with your physician if you had a terminal disease? Why or why not?

3. Although Patrick was young, his story shows us the reality of people living with chronic, yet ultimately terminal illnesses. What did you learn from Patrick's experience?

4

The Heart of The Matter

By the time I met Walter Atkins, he was already dead. His body lay in the emergency room trauma bay, unmoved since they'd first wheeled him in from the ambulance. The ER doctors had acted fast, but the CT scan of his head had come back showing a devastating brain bleed.

"Young kid," Dr. Baxter said, shaking his head solemnly. He was the ER doctor who had called me to evaluate Walter for the ICU. "It's terrible, he probably ruptured an aneurysm. Parents found him down in his apartment. The scan shows that he's herniating." He pulled up the x-ray images on the viewer.

Herniating: the black cloud of neurology. The worst-case scenario. The precursor to brain death. Dr. Baxter navigated the CT images screen for me to view. The two sides of the grey brain images appeared aligned next to each other, with each subsequent image showing more and more "white stuff."

"Is that blood?" a voice shot out from behind me. Startled, I turned my head and saw that a medical student had snuck up on us. He was wearing scrubs under his short white coat, so I assumed he was a student rotating in the ER.

"Hi, Chris," Dr. Baxter said. "Yeah, unfortunately, it is. All the white you see here is blood in his brain. You can see how the blood is actually pushing the brain tissue over to the side, pressing the brain up against the side of his skull."

Chris made a face. "Not good," he muttered.

"Actually, Chris, since you just got here, this is a good case for you to follow. Dr. Van Scoy, do you mind if Chris hangs out with you for awhile?"

I didn't. "No problem. Call me L. J." I held out my hand to shake Chris's hand, then turned to introduce him to Arvin, my neurology resident.

Dr. Baxter said, "L. J. is the ICU fellow, so you can follow her until the patient goes up to the unit. We don't have much else going on down here right now, so this should be more educational for you."

I took one last look at the pictures of my new patient's brain, and pressed my lips together. It was time to get started.

"Okay, Arvin, why don't you present the case to us, and then we'll all go see him together. We've seen his imaging, but let's hear the story." I moved toward the chart rack.

Arvin snapped into action, a contrast from the stillness he'd exuded while looking at the image. He straightened himself up so much that he seemed to grow two inches taller and began.

"The patient is a twenty-nine year old white male with no past medical history who was found on the ground in his apartment by his mother earlier this afternoon. She had come over to his apartment after she heard that he hadn't come to work and he didn't return his calls." He paused, his formality fading. "Uh, that's really it. He had no past medical history, so . . ."

"He's never had any surgery?" I inquired.

"No, never," Arvin answered.

"Medications?"

Arvin shook his head.

"Recent illnesses?"

"Nope."

"Totally healthy?"

"Yeah, I asked his parents. No medical problems," Arvin confirmed.

"So, what was his exam like?" The question was just a formality, since I would be examining the patient myself, but I also wanted to test Arvin to know how thorough and accurate he had been in assessing the patient.

"Well, he is on the ventilator and isn't taking any spontaneous breaths. His pupils are nonreactive, and he doesn't withdraw to any painful stimuli. No gag reflex. No deep tendon reflexes. No oculocephalics. Nothing," Arvin said.

"So, from what you're telling me, he's dead."

"Yeah, I believe he is," Arvin answered.

"What about the rest of his exam: heart, lungs?"

Chris looked at me as if I had six heads. He was perplexed, and I knew why, but I wanted to give him the opportunity to hear the answer before I explained.

"Heart and lungs were normal. Normal heart sounds. Regular heart rate. No murmurs. No arrhythmias. Lungs were clear on both sides." Arvin rattled off his findings, and I watched as Chris furrowed his brow in confusion.

Interrupting Arvin as he was telling me about the abdominal exam, I asked Chris what was the matter.

"Well, didn't we just say he is dead? But, uh, now we're saying the heart exam was normal," Chris asked.

"He's brain dead. It's different," Arvin explained.

"Well, actually, no," I interrupted again. "Dead is dead. But what you mean is he did not have a cardiac death. He had a brain death. Well, that's what it seems. We have to go see him to be sure, but if what Arvin is saying is correct, then yes, he is dead even though his heart is beating."

"Oh," Chris said. He opened his mouth to ask another question, but shut it again and looked over at me.

"We'll get there." I motioned for the guys to follow me. "Let's go see him first, and then we'll talk about all the details. If he has herniated, then it's very likely that he is already brain dead. But if not, we'll have to act fast. Was neurosurgery called?"

Dr. Baxter overheard my question and answered from the across the nursing station, "I called Dr. Anteas. He's reviewing the films now."

"What about family?" I asked. "Do they know what's going on?

"I didn't tell them too much, except that it doesn't look good, and we are having the neurosurgeons look at his film," Dr. Baxter answered.

"Great," I turned to Arvin, "Lead the way."

We all went into ER Room 2, where the curtain was drawn around Walter's bed. Underneath the curtain, I could see four feet, probably the parents', who were sitting on two chairs facing the bed.

Arvin pulled open the curtain, and I was taken aback by the couple in front of me, so stoic on their small plastic chairs. Typically, when I walk into a room, my eyes first dart to the monitors before addressing the patient or family, just to be sure everything is stable. But in this room, the stillness of these two people drew my eyes to them and only them. I didn't even look at the patient; the parents' faces said it all. They were pale, tear-stained, and distraught. I knew that the person who needed the most help was, in fact, not the patient, but his parents. They were in shock.

"This is Dr. Van Scoy," Arvin began and gestured to me. "She's the intensive care fellow."

"Hello," I said softly, holding out my hand for the husband and wife. Each took turns shaking my hand in silence, barely looking up from the floor. "And this is Chris, one of our medical students.

"I'm just going to examine your son, and then we'll talk about what we're going to do from here, all right?" They nodded ever so slightly, and I headed over to the stretcher.

A ventilator tube jutted from Walter's clean-shaven jaw. His eyes were shut and his skin was flushed with color, hardly the way anyone would expect a dead man to look. Placing my hand on his shins, I checked for warmth. Yes, blood was perfusing to his legs. Next, his arms: same thing. His healthy heart was pumping blood to his extremities. On to the monitors: his heart rate was 80 beats per minute and his blood pressure a perfect 120/80. The ventilator sounds whirred without any alarms, and I could hear the air whoosh in and out of his perfectly normal lungs. His body was as sound as my own, but his brain was destroyed.

The rest of the exam proceeded quickly, and I moved slowly and methodically so as not to disturb his body in any way. The room was silent, and my every motion felt like a tidal wave amidst the stillness. I tried to keep my attention solely on Walter, even though I could feel Arvin's, Chris's, and Walter's parents' eyes on me, watching me intently.

Arvin's report of the physical exam had been spot on; it was completely normal. Now it was time to test brain function. Before I started, I glanced over at the drips on the pole above Walter's head. Only IV fluids were being infused—no medications. Walter's body didn't require anything else, and we were giving him the fluid since he couldn't eat or drink and probably hadn't for quite some time.

"Did he get any meds?" I asked Arvin.

Arvin nodded. "When they intubated him, they gave him some sedative and fentanyl."

"Right." I flashed a look at Arvin that I hoped said *damn it*. The medications would alter the neurologic exam that I was about to perform, making any definitive decisions based on the exam impossible. Sedatives and narcotics affect the neural reflexes in such a way that you can't actually declare someone officially brain dead until those medications completely wore off. That would take about six hours. And for any family, that's a long time to wait without knowing if your loved one is dead or alive.

Gently lifting Walter's eyelids, I held my penlight in my other hand. "I'm going to shine a light in your eyes, Walter." This was more for his parents' benefit than for his, as he couldn't hear me. The pupils didn't move when exposed to the light, as they should if the reflex was functioning. Next, I took out a swab of cotton from the cabinet next to the stretcher and twirled its end into a fine point. Again, I lifted his eyelid and dabbed the cotton tip onto the surface of his eyeball. There was no reflex for him to blink. He was 0 for 2. Next, I checked his oculocephalic reflex, what we call "doll's eyes." I took Walter's head in my hands and moved his head from side to side, watching his eyes. They remained fixed, his gaze not moving as I turned his head. Not good. Next, I looked at the ventilator's rate, set at 16. Walter was breathing at a rate of 16, which told me that the machine was doing all the breathing since Walter's brain wasn't triggering any extra breaths. Since the brain tells your lungs to breathe, even when someone is on a breathing machine they might breathe over the vent, which we call "over breathing." Over breathing is a good sign. It means that the brain is stimulating extra breaths, independent of the ventilator. But in Walter's case, there were no extra breaths. I reached over to the tube jutting out of his mouth and jostled it ever so slightly, to see if I could trigger Walter to cough or gag from the stimulation in the back of his throat. Nothing.

A glance over to Arvin and we silently agreed: he was gone. There was still one test I had left to do, which involved squirting cold water into his ear, but I decided to defer that until later, considering we'd have to repeat the same exam after the medications wore off. My time would be better spent talking to the neurosurgeons and then initiating what was going to be a rather difficult discussion with Walter's mom and dad.

No sooner had Arvin, Chris and I walked out of Walter's room than Dr. Anteas had called in to the ER.

"Hi Dr. Anteas," I said. "This is L. J."

"Oh, hey, L. J. How's it going?" he asked cheerily.

"It's going." My standard reply. "Did you take a look at these films?"

"Yeah, from what I hear, he has no brainstem reflexes."

"Uh huh. I just saw him and I wasn't able to elicit any reflex, but he did get some ativan and opioids during his intubation, so I can't say for sure."

"Okay, I already spoke with Dr. Conn, and he is willing to take him to the IR suite and take a look to see if there is anything he can coil."

"Really?" I didn't hide the shock in my voice. IR stood for interventional radiology, which meant they were considering just that: an intervention. "At least its something we can try. Are you considering taking him to surgery? I just assumed that he's too far gone for that."

"He probably is, but there's a possibility we could put in a drain, but we'll have to see what happens in IR."

"Sounds like a plan." This was more hopeful, since he thought there was a possibility for an intervention.

"I'm on my way in," Dr. Anteas said. "I'll see you in a few minutes."

Arvin, I could see, had already turned to the computer to place the orders while I made a few phone calls to procure a bed for Walter in the ICU. Once the calls were made, I turned to Chris.

"Confused yet?" I asked him with a smile.

"Completely and totally."

Once the admission paperwork and calls were completed, I decided I had been stalling long enough. We had to talk to Walter's family. Arvin was working diligently on his admission orders, so I motioned to Chris to come along with me for The Discussion. There would need to be a lot of explanations, both for the family and for Chris, who thankfully wasn't bombarding me with questions just yet. Perhaps he could sense my angst. Although I've had many of these conversations with families in the past, it wasn't very common that the patient was an otherwise healthy young man, particularly one who was just a year younger than me. How would Walter's parents feel getting this information from someone so close to his age?

When we returned to Walter's room, his family was exactly as I had left them. "How are you doing?" I asked this as an icebreaker and was met with silent shrugs. But it was a start. I looked around for another chair but didn't see any within the immediate area. This was going to be a different experience for me as well; I didn't commonly have discussions like this in the emergency room. Most of the time I preferred to have the patients settled into the unit before making any firm judgment or recommendations. But in this case, I was making an exception. It was going to take a long time for them to process the information I was going to give them and usually it took families many hours, even days, for the reality to sink in. The sooner we started the conversation, the better.

"Well, let me start off by saying that I'm terribly sorry to meet you under these circumstances. In case you forgot, my name is Dr. Van Scoy, and I'm one of the critical care fellows. The ER called me so that we can get Walter upstairs to the intensive care unit," I said, the words rolling off my tongue. It was my typical intro that I resorted to when I was otherwise at a loss for words.

Walter's mother reached out her hand. "I'm Ilene and this is my husband Jake."

Jake looked at the ground but nodded his head in a feeble hello.

"I'm not exactly sure how much Dr. Baxter has already explained to you, so why don't you summarize for me what you've understood so far and we'll pick it up from there," I said. It was as good as a place as any to start, and with any luck, they may tell me that they already knew he was probably brain dead. That would make my job a lot easier.

"Well, we know he had a big bleed in his head and that it doesn't look very good, but other than that, we don't know how this happened or if the surgeons are going to take him to surgery or what." Ilene picked up speed as she went. "I just don't understand what happened."

"Okay, well, you're exactly right," I began. "Walter does have a lot of blood in his brain right now. Whether it's the result of some sort of fall or trauma or if it was a brain aneurysm that ruptured, we just don't know yet."

As I spoke, a terrible thought crept into my head. I didn't know if he had a urine drug screen or an alcohol level when he arrived. This would be much worse if it turned out that the bleed was after a drunken fall or a cocaine binge. I hoped that wasn't the case, for his parent's sake, and made a mental note to myself to remember to make sure the ER had sent off those tests.

Trying not to look or seem distracted, I continued in my monologue.

"The cause of the bleed isn't terribly relevant at this point, although if it was an aneurysm, the interventional radiologist doctors may be able to place a coil inside the aneurysm in order to plug it up and contain the bleeding or prevent another rupture. The problem with that is, there has been a lot of brain damage already, and the coil can't do anything about damage already done, but it's something we're looking into."

A look of hope crossed Jake's otherwise expressionless face, so much that I began backpedalling immediately.

"Unfortunately, though, there is a chance that Walter's brain is already so badly damaged that it may not even be functioning any more, which is called brain death," I said it as bluntly as I could, the words sounding vulgar as they resonated in the room. But it had to be said. I paused for some kind of reaction, got none and thus continued, slipping into formalities.

"Earlier, when we were examining Walter, we did some very simple tests that help us to determine whether the brain is actually functioning. Simple things like when I flashed the light in his eyes to see if his pupils would get smaller or when I moved the breathing tube around to see if he would gag. And, well, unfortunately, he didn't respond," I said. Again, I paused and was met with blank stares. *Keep going, L. J.,* I told myself. *Keep going.*

"We have him hooked up to the ventilator, not, not because his lungs are sick, but because his brain isn't telling him to breathe, which is another sign that his brain is not functioning. So, so he's fully dependent on the life support." I was beginning to stutter and looked over at Chris for just a moment, just to have someplace else to divert my eyes, but his face was as blank and dismal as Walter's parents'.

"What are you saying, doc, that he has brain damage?" Jake's voice cracked on *damage*.

"Well, yes. He most definitely has brain damage, but I guess what I'm trying to say is that I'm very concerned that his brain is at risk of dying completely, if it hasn't already," I answered. "The most worrisome thing is that his brain is herniating."

I paused to see if there was any reaction to the word. There wasn't.

"So, what that means, is that, well . . . you know that the brain is encased by the skull and there are holes in the skull in different places. So, what can happen is that when there is increased pressure within the skull cavity or within the brain, like, for example, if there is suddenly a lot of blood in the brain, then the brain tissue itself can actually push, or herniate, through the holes in the skull." I tried to illustrate by curving my fingers into a circle and pushing my other hand through the makeshift hole. It was graphic but necessary.

"So, the fact that this is happening, and we can see it on the CT scan, is a very ominous sign that he may, in fact, have brain death. The problem is that we can't really know for sure until the medications that he was given when he was put on the breathing machine have worn off, which is going to take several hours."

"Okay, so we wait and see then," Ilene said, nodding her head while wringing her hands together. I knew that the only thing they probably retained from my whole dialogue was that we couldn't really know for sure yet. But that was okay. They'd heard it all once through, and you have to start somewhere.

"Yes, we're going to wait and see. In the meantime, I already spoke to the neurosurgeons and the interventional radiologists, and they are going to talk to you about possibly doing that coiling procedure I explained before." The looks on their faces made me stop. I could see they could barely remember what I had said seconds before, which under the circumstances was not surprising at all. I'd say it as many times as I had to, plus I had the benefit of having Chris as an audience, so I could use the opportunity to teach him something, too.

"What they do is, they inject some dye into a vein so they can look at the blood vessels in the brain and watch the blood flow. The dye makes a 'road map' of the blood vessels in the brain. They can then see if there is an aneurysm, which is what we think may have been the cause of all of this."

Ilene asked, "What exactly is an aneurysm?"

Oy, I thought to myself, feeling bad that I hadn't explained that earlier. Talking with patients can be difficult, because I don't want to choose words that non-medical people wouldn't understand, but I don't want to sound condescending by simplifying things too much. Families get annoyed either way, but I was lucky that Ilene was smart enough to admit that she didn't understand.

"An aneurysm is like a balloon, or a pouch that forms alongside a blood vessel. It bulges out from a weakness in the side of a blood vessel, and as it bulges, the wall stretches and can rupture. If Walter has an aneurysm, they may be able to thread a coil inside the balloon to plug it up and stop the bleeding. But, again, a coil can't do anything about the damage that's already been done," I told them.

They began nodding, and I could see that they understood. I waited for them to wrap their heads around the concept, so I kept quiet while they digested it.

Jake finally asked, "When are they going to do this procedure?"

"As soon as possible, I presume. The interventional radiologist, Dr. Conn will probably come talk to you and get you to sign a consent form and he'll give you the specifics. In the meantime, I'm getting a room ready for him in the ICU."

Ilene tried to get the full picture: "And is this instead of doing surgery?"

"Well, that's really a question for the neurosurgeons and the radiologists." I hedged because I wasn't sure, and I didn't want to mention the possibility of the drain until I knew if Dr. Anteas was going to pursue that route. So, I was grateful when I saw Dr. Anteas enter the room. He was wearing his bright green scrubs, ready for action in the OR if the situation required it. Having him there gave me a tinge of hope. Maybe I was wrong, and there was something we could do for Walter. As Dr. Anteas introduced himself to Walter's parents, I glanced back over to Walter's ventilator. Still no extra breaths. Still no signs of life.

"I think I get it now," Chris said as we left the room. We had excused ourselves while Dr. Anteas examined Walter and interviewed his parents.

"Get what?" I asked, realizing I still hadn't really explained anything about what was happening to Chris.

"How he can be dead yet still have a heart beat and a blood pressure," he said.

I smiled. He had probably been pondering this during the whole dialogue that had just happened. It was confusing as hell. "Tell me," I encouraged.

"The heart has its own innervation, so even when the brain dies, the heart can still beat. It has automaticity," he said proudly.

"Yep. You got it," I said. "Don't you just love anatomy?"

He chuckled. "Not really."

"I was never very good at anatomy either," I admitted. "The fact that the heart has cells capable of generating their own electrical impulses to stimulate a heart beat is pretty amazing. Especially since that means the heart can beat even without a brain. It makes things difficult, though. Lay people aren't used to thinking about life and death in terms of anatomy."

"Yeah, I mean, he doesn't look dead," Chris said.

"Well, he probably is, but we'll know for sure soon enough," I said. "In the meantime, I better give Dr. York a call and let him know what's going on."

Dr. York was the ICU attending on tonight. He was my supervisor, reviewing all my work and decisions. Just as I was overseeing the medical students, interns and residents, Dr. York was overseeing me, right up the chain of command.

Dr. York heard all the particulars of this case and approved. "Sounds good. Well, it sounds awful, but the plan sounds good.

"Once the meds wear off, start the brain death protocol," he instructed. "What time do you think the second formal exam will be?"

"Probably early tomorrow morning." The protocol involved two formal neurologic exams without any medications on board, and those exams had to be about eight hours apart. I glanced at the clock, then counted the hours on my fingers. "Around eight or nine in the morning."

"All right," Dr. York said. "Let me know if anything changes."

"You got it," I said. "Have a good night. Hope I won't talk to you again!"

"Yeah, I hope not," he answered with a laugh. If we had to speak again, that would mean someone was very sick and I needed help or that there was another admission to the unit. When on night call, the less you had to talk to your attending, the slower the night and the more sleep you got. Unfortunate for Walter, I didn't expect too much to come up.

An hour later, Arvin and I were back upstairs in the unit reviewing Walter's labs, awaiting his arrival to the unit from IR. His labs were all normal, there was no alcohol or drugs in his system, and so it was looking more and more like this was probably a ruptured aneurysm. Arvin and I were scouring the computer system to see if Walter had been to our hospital before and if there were any clues to what had happened lurking in his old records. We had just given up when Dr. Anteas came into the unit.

I looked up, not expecting much. "Any news?"

"No, he's in IR now. I just came up to check on another patient while we wait."

Arvin asked, "Do you think you might take Walter to the OR?"

Dr. Anteas shook his head. "I doubt it."

"But, isn't it at least something we can try?"

Sitting down on the edge of the computer table with his legs dangling off the side, Dr. Anteas stated the sad truth. "You know, there are worse things than dying. It's much easier for us to do the wrong thing than it is to do the right thing.

"If he's not already brain dead, I could take Walter to the OR and drill a hole in his head and place a drain inside his brain and maybe, *maybe*, save his life. Maybe by taking the blood out and the pressure off I might prevent him from herniating to the point of brain death. But, then what? The question you have to ask yourself is what are you left with *then*, and are you prepared to deal with the consequences?"

Arvin and I sat silent.

"I mean, you'll be left with a twenty-nine-year-old kid, healthy as can be, except he is in a permanent coma. He'll never wake up. He'll never open eyes or say hello to his family, or even know they're there. He'll exist within some institution, a hospital, nursing home, whatever, for the rest of his life. He'll get infections and have a feeding tube. He'll have a rectal tube and a Foley forever. He'll move only when the nurses turn him. He'll get bedsores. He'll have no quality of life, no awareness. And his family will be left with a son whose body is alive, but that's it."

Dr. Anteas's eyes were alive with emotion. "So, like I said, there are worse things than dying."

It wasn't long before we got the call. No flow. There was no blood flow to either side the brain. Zero. In a way, it was a blessing. I now had definitive evidence of what we suspected from the very beginning. Walter was dead. He was dead the moment he arrived in the ER, but the fact that his heart continued to beat made the situation . . . sticky. Not uncertain, but sticky. There wasn't any doubt that Walter was dead, but the fact that his body was warm, you could feel his pulses, and the ventilator made his chest rise up and down with each delivered breath presented a picture of a man in a deep coma, not the picture of a dead man. Our job as the medical team was going to be explaining the difference between brain death and cardiac death to Ilene and Jake Atkins and to tell them that Walter was already gone.

"Go ahead and call Gift of Life," I instructed Arvin. "I don't know if he's an organ donor or not, but it's time to make the call."

Arvin nodded and dialled. It was too late for Walter, but maybe there was someone who could be saved.

Once Walter's body and his family were settled in the room, I turned to Arvin. Dr. Anteas had gotten called away to another emergency in the ER, and now, rather than wait for him to return, I had decided to relay the news.

"Do you want to lead the talk?" I offered.

"Not particularly," Arvin admitted. "I'd rather just listen."

"Okay," I said. I should have insisted that Arvin lead the discussion, but the truth was, I wanted to do it myself. I had already started the discussion earlier and so it was probably less confusing for Ilene and Jake if they had one doctor as their point person. "You'll be the one here through the night, though, so you should come with me. They need to get to know you, too."

Arvin agreed and we headed toward Walter's new room.

On the way, I stopped abruptly and turned to Arvin.

"Don't mention organ donation," I told him sternly. "Gift of Life doesn't want the physicians taking care of him to bring it up. They prefer to bring it up themselves."

Arvin nodded. "Yeah, I know."

State law mandates that for every death, the organ donation agency has to be notified, regardless of whether or not the patient was a candidate for organ donation or not. But bringing up the concept of organ donation was not the job of the physicians taking care of the patient. We had to focus on Walter and his brain, not his healthy organs.

"Hi there," I said as I entered the room. Ilene and Jake were seated by the windowsill. Ilene was talking on her cell phone, and Jake was seated quietly, watching the monitors as they displayed Walter's heart rate and blood pressure.

Ilene ended her call and turned to say hello.

We exchanged pleasantries as I walked to Walter's bedside, where I rubbed his leg gently over the blankets. My eyes stayed on Jake and Ilene, trying to gauge how they were coping. Ilene seemed exhausted and her eyes were red with fatigue and tears. Jake was harder to read. He remained the same stoic statue, staring at the ground whenever I tried to meet his eyes.

"I just got the result from the procedure, and when they tried to measure the blood flow to Walter's brain, well, I'm really sorry to say that there was not any flow." I stopped to take a breath and let that sink in before I dealt the next blow. "That means that there is no blood going to his brain, which means that he has brain death."

Jake broke down first, burying his head in his hands, moaning and mumbling some words I couldn't understand. Ilene sobbed and turned her head into Jake's shoulder.

Arvin stood silently next to me and we looked at each other with sad looks, both of us feeling helpless and useless. I said the only thing I could: "I'm so sorry."

As they began to grieve, I struggled with how long to wait before moving the conversation forward into discussions of policy and protocol. They had to know what would happen next, to get on with the inevitable reality that we would be taking away the machines since Walter was dead, but I didn't want to rush it.

Legally, I could have declared Walter brain dead and filled out his death certificate right then. The result of the flow study combined with the neurologic exam was definitive evidence. But since the flow study wasn't a test we commonly ordered, the hospital had a policy, "the brain death protocol," to help us dot the Is and cross the Ts. The policy was just wishy-washy enough that it left it up to my clinical judgment whether there needed to be an observation period before declaring brain death. There was no blanket statement, no magic formula; instead, we had a series of recommendations based on ethical, legal, and moral principles established within medical societies.

An observation period during which two full neurologic exams are performed, approximately eight hours apart is sometimes initiated, usually in the absence of other testing. After the second exam, if the exam reveals brain death, the patient is declared deceased. The patient is then removed from the ventilator and in the absence of oxygen, the heart eventually stops beating.

In Walter's case, though, I didn't need a protocol. There was no uncertainty here because I had a flow study showing zero blood flow to the brain, but there certainly wasn't much harm in extending the brain death protocol to its final detail. Although an observation period was not necessary in Walter's case, I favored an observation period, as did Dr. York, knowing that the extra time would allow Ilene and Jake a little extra time to process, grieve and to say goodbye.

And so, against my scientific instincts, I chose not to declare Walter dead, but instead began to explain the "brain death protocol." With Arvin standing solemnly at my side, I told Jake and Ilene that in the morning, around eight o'clock, Dr. York would arrive and we would all meet together and perform one final exam. If it was consistent with brain death, as we expected it would be, the machines would be removed from Walter's body.

My words were halting and hard. They continued to cry and attempted to console one another. Gently, I offered my own condolences, and left the clock ticking behind me.

By the time I made it to Walter's room the next day, Dr. Greenberg, the neurology attending, was examining Walter with Arvin. Jake and Ilene were not there, but I noticed their bags on the window ledge, so I knew they hadn't gone far, probably to get some coffee. There were crumpled blankets over the chairs, so I presumed they had spent the night at Walter's side.

"Good morning." I greeted Dr. Greenberg as he moved Walter's head from side to side, observing his eye movements, or lack thereof.

"Hi," Dr. Greenberg answered, looking up from his exam. "Did you admit him last night?"

Dr. Greenberg wasn't my attending, but I suddenly got nervous that I was about to get ridiculed for admitting a dead man to the intensive care unit and furthermore for keeping his body alive through the night. He was in his mid-fifties and significantly higher up than me in the hospital food chain.

"Yes," I said.

"Have you met the family?" he asked me.

"Yes, I spoke with them for a while last night." I was unsure if Dr. Greenberg was upset with me or if he was just being matter of fact. "I explained the brain death protocol to them late last night, so they sort of know what's going on, but I still think we should review everything with them again, now that's its morning."

"Sure." His tone was warmer now. Maybe he was happy that the worst part of the job had already been done. His stress level seemed to decrease once he knew that the initial discussion had already been done.

"I'm happy to meet with them, too, if you'd like. Who is the ICU attending?"

Relieved that he wasn't angry, I was grateful for his offer. "That would be great. Dr. York is the attending, and I'm going to arrange a meeting between him and the family, so if you'd like to come, I'm sure that would be helpful." I always felt that the more different specialists at a family meeting, the better. It made the family feel like we were covering all our bases, and in the situation of brain death, it was probably comforting for them to also hear the dismal news from a neurologist. It wasn't really necessary, considering any physician can diagnose and declare brain death, but I thought it would be helpful to have a neurologist to answer any questions Ilene and Jake might have, particularly since we would be removing the ventilator once the final exam was performed. I was pleased Dr. Greenberg volunteered to be there.

"Just page me when you are meeting, and I'll be there."

He left the room and Arvin, being a future neurologist, fell into step right behind him, leaving me alone with Walter for the first time. It was hard to see him, so young and so much like me. I thought about his young, healthy body with its non-functioning brain and shook away the thoughts of whether Walter's healthy organs might save someone else's life.

When it was time for the meeting, I led the Atkinses into the conference room, and they sat down without a word. Since the residents were all still preparing their morning progress notes, I was the youngest doctor in the room, so I said nothing and waited for my seniors to begin the meeting. Dr. York began by introducing himself and Dr. Greenberg and then summarized all the events that had transpired thus far. As he spoke, I let my eyes and thoughts wander. On one side of the conference table sat Walter's parents, wearing the same clothing from the night before, looking tired and shattered. I had memorized Jake and Ilene's stoic faces since we had first met, and this morning they looked no different. Now, with Dr. York leading the conversation instead of me, I had a chance to really study them. They were a timid couple; in fact, they rarely spoke, and I wondered if this was who they were or if it was their grief disguised as shyness.

On the other side of the table were the three of us doctors, a strange collection of characters, I had to admit. First, there was me, the youngest in the room. I was the only one wearing a white coat, which, in this sort of meeting, I relied upon to serve as a reminder to myself that I was at work, performing a job. I was painfully aware that my age was essentially the same as Walter's, and for this I felt like an imposter. My white coat served as a barrier, keeping my emotional self at a distance from the family members seated in front of me.

Then, there was Dr. York, who was in his mid-forties, an energetic ICU doctor who dressed the part in his blue scrubs and shaggy hair. As he spoke, his words were cushioned by his experience in critical care, and I envied his ease with this. His age put a certain emphasis behind everything he said, and I noticed that the Atkinses seemed to listen to him with a different intentness than they did when I had spoken with them.

Lastly, sitting on the end was the neurology attending, Dr. Greenberg, wearing a three-piece suit. His tie had a silver and blue pattern that popped from his charcoal gray sport coat. No doubt he had office hours later on this morning, but the contrast of his attire from Dr. York's and mine made him stand out.

As Dr. York finished his recap, I noticed the Jake and Ilene's demeanor begin to change. Maybe it was because of hearing the events from Dr. York, who was older and more authoritative looking than me, or maybe because it was their second or third time hearing the terrible truth of Walter's condition, but I began to see their faces change ever so slightly from a state of shock, to a state of intense sadness. Jake Atkins looked over at Dr. Greenberg after Dr. York finished speaking, prompting Dr. Greenberg to speak.

"I agree with everything you just heard," he said, obviously picking up on the need for even more confirmation. "I examined your son earlier this morning, and he didn't have any of the basic brainstem reflexes that are compatible with life."

Upon hearing the words from Dr. Greenberg, Jake broke down. As he and his wife cried, the three of us on the other side of the table sat quietly and respectfully, patiently waiting for whatever was going to happen next. Silence was important in situations like this—that was lesson number one from medical school—yet our silence stood out to me like a flashing light against the Atkins' cries and sobs.

Dr. York was the one who finally spoke first.

"We're going to perform the second neurologic exam and, based on the result, we'll then begin the process of removing the machine," he said. "Is there anyone else you'd like to come to the hospital before we do that?"

"No," Ilene managed, her voice high pitched and shaking.

Jake leaned forward. "When you remove the machines, what will happen then? He just . . . dies?"

"No, Mr. Atkins," Dr. York said, "he is already dead. When we take away the ventilator, his body will stop getting oxygen, and eventually his heart will stop beating. Right now, the heart is still working because we are feeding it with oxygen, and it has its own power supply, independent of the brain. But, removing the machine isn't allowing him to die, because he's already gone. The only thing that will change is that his heart will no longer beat."

Jake Atkins looked at all of us as we sat there nodding our heads in agreement. Ilene put her head down on the table, burying her face in her arms. I pitied them as they tried to understand how their son's heart could beat as we were telling them he was already gone. It was confusing even to me, and this wasn't the first nor would it be the last brain death case I'd be involved in.

Science, religion, and philosophy were colliding in my head. How do we define death? What is it to be alive? Why is a beating heart not a sign of life? My instincts nagged me otherwise. I thought about how Chris had been so confused in the ER, and he was a medical student, with medical training. Yet, he had to "figure out" what death meant. Here was the conundrum I had foreseen back when I first viewed Walter's brain images in the ER, dreading the tasks ahead, including explaining it all in a way that a family, this family, the Atkinses, could understand.

Knowing and believing in science and medicine has always been enough for me, and in my medical mind, brain death is just another type of death. Medicine and science have gone to great lengths pinpointing the definition of death. I stretched my mind to try to humanize my definition by taking myself out of the scientific world I live in and morphing it into a more intuitive one. Perhaps, I thought, it might not be enough to simply leave it at that. If it were my husband, or son, or friend, or parent lying in that bed instead of Walter, would I truly feel and believe that he was dead, with his flushed face, warm skin, and beating heart?

"But will he feel pain?" Ilene asked as I shook my thoughts to the back of my mind and focused on the room again.

"No, he won't have any pain," Dr. York said. "His brain can't perceive pain."

"When is the next exam?" Jake asked.

Dr. York looked over at me.

"Whenever you're ready," I said.

Dr. York and Dr. Greenberg stood up and offered their hands and final condolences to the Atkinses. Jake and Ilene rose as well.

"There's no rush," I assured them as the attendings left the room. "Take all the time you like with Walter, and then let the nurse know when you're ready for me to come in and do the exam."

"Okay, thank you." Ilene passed me as I held the door open for her and Jake. I waited behind so they wouldn't feel my presence following them to the room. In the meantime, I figured I'd check in with the residents and see how things were going in preparation for morning rounds.

Back in the unit, I searched for my resident teams to see if there was anything I could do to help them get ready for rounds, but they were all scurrying around like a bunch of flies trapped in a jar. Rather than slowing them down, I decided to flip through some of the charts as I waited for my summons from Walter's parents. As I opened the first chart, I saw the Gift of Life representative paging through Walter's medical record. I stared at the chart pages as I flipped, not really reading what was written on the pages as they passed. I was too distracted, so it was a relief when I got the summons twenty minutes later from Walter's nurse, Joe, who motioned to me from across the room. It was time.

As I stood over Walter, shining my penlight in his eye, I was painfully aware that I was only going through the motions. I repeated the same maneuvers I had done the evening before, this time with my attending in the room to make it even more official. For completion sake, I even did the cold caloric test, in which I injected cold water into Walter's ears to observe if he had nystagmus, or eye movements in response to the water. I did five or six maneuvers, and all confirmed brain death.

"Time of death, 8:42 a.m.," I said quietly, more for myself so I would remember the time for the death certificate. I took a step back from his bed and looked at my dead patient. It was approximately fifteen hours since I had first met Walter, and, sadly, nothing had changed since the moment he had arrived, except that his parents had begun the process of accepting that their son was dead.

We removed the machines ten minutes later. Jake and Ilene had declined organ donation for religious reasons, so there was no reason to wait. Dr. York and Dr. Greenberg had moved on to begin their daily rounds, and I was left to withdraw the machines with the nurse and respiratory therapist. The Atkinses had decided to stay outside the room while we removed the ventilator, making the process a lot quicker since I didn't need to explain what I was doing. Joe, the nurse, suctioned Walter's mouth out to prevent any extra drool or secretions from sliding out along with the ventilator tubing and messing up his hospital gown. As Joe did the suctioning, the respiratory therapist, Nancy, prepared the tube so it would be easily withdrawn by removing the straps and deflating the ventilator cuff. With a swift move, she pulled the tube out of Walter's mouth and Joe did his cleanup with the suction catheter. The ventilator alarms screamed until Nancy was able to reach over and slap the silence button as if it was the snooze button on her alarm clock. The whole process took about ten seconds, and other than the brief alarms, the atmosphere in the room was quiet and sombre.

"Can I bring them in?" I asked Joe.

"I'll get them," he answered and slipped out the door, anxious to get out of the room.

I went over to the monitor and looked at its screen. His heart rate was a perfect 70 beats per minute, with the EKG tracing showing a picture perfect rhythm. His blood pressure was equally perfect. His oxygen level read 99 percent. I reached up and switched off the screen so that when Jake and Ilene came back in the room, they wouldn't see his vital signs. They were just numbers at this point, perfect numbers, in fact, but with no meaning.

The Atkinses came in just as I switched off the monitor, and the silent room was suddenly filled with tears and sobs. Nancy, Joe, and I quietly left the room to allow them time alone with Walter. We congregated in the nursing station, watching the remote monitor of Walter's vital signs. Without the ventilator, Walter's body had no way of getting oxygen and so his oxygen level had already dropped to 90 percent. His heart was still beating, and we could see that his heart rate and blood pressure had barely changed. I looked through the window leading into Walter's room and saw his mother with her head resting on Walter's chest as she sobbed. Jake wasn't in my view, so I assumed he was seated on a chair further back in the room.

Joe and I sat vigilantly by the monitor, not talking much as we watched Walter's oxygen levels drop. Nancy had already moved on to administer a breathing treatment to another patient in need, but neither Joe nor I had anywhere better to be. So, we just sat and watched as Walter's numbers gradually crept from perfect to less so. His heart rate slowed and his blood pressure dropped until finally, his heart stopped altogether. It took about fifteen minutes from the time we took the ventilator away until his heart stopped completely.

As I opened the door to Walter's room, his mom lifted her head from Walter's chest and turned towards me.

She wailed, "He's gone, isn't he?"

I hesitated, holding back the urge to reinforce the fact that he had gone long ago, but that the electrical energy of the heart had stopped. But I knew that the beating heart was far too symbolic of life to explain away with science.

"Yes, his heart just stopped beating."

"I know," she cried, "I heard it. I heard the whole thing. I heard it when it stopped."

Jake Atkins held his head low, crying full, wet tears. And for just a moment, I too felt what Jake and Ilene Atkins felt, that Walter had died just then, just in that moment, with the silencing of his heart.

"We're all outside if you need anything," I managed to say, surprised at my own thoughts as I backed out the door, retreating back into the world of science and medicine.

* * *

The diagnosis of brain death can be either a blessing or a curse. When it's happening to your loved one, it's always a curse. Yet, underlying all the horror of the fact that someone you care about is dead, I'm always mindful of the hidden blessing that I've come to observe from interacting with families like Walter's. And when I say hidden, I mean completely invisible to anyone but an outsider not personally engaged in the horror of the situation as it unfolds. However, it lingers quietly in the background. It may seem inconceivable, but there is a small glimmer of light that is offered to these families as they suffer upon hearing the finality of the diagnosis of brain death. They are spared the burden of making the difficult choices in a hopeless situation. Their loved one is already gone. There is no decision to be made.

Brain death often occurs unexpectedly, either after an accident, such as the case of actress Natasha Richardson who famously had brain death after a seemingly minor skiing accident, or from a severe stroke or swelling of the brain for various medical reasons. Rarely are families prepared for the devastating news that hijacks their lives.

While families like Walter's tensely await word from the doctors, praying to hear that their loved one has not in fact already died, still others subconsciously or perhaps consciously wish for their loved ones to go peacefully, on their own accord, rather than continuing a prolonged life without awareness.

It is these latter families, whose loved ones linger in an uncertain state, with stories that are equally tragic, equally gut-wrenching, that leave me to wonder if they are the victims of something which may be far worse than death of a loved one. They are the victims of an uncertain yet looming choice, whether or not to continue to press on while the brain still lives, yet has been permanently injured.

Too often I have watched as these families are left with the burden of making a decision about whether to forego life support, or perhaps eliminate a feeding tube. Their loved ones may reside in a state of what we call "anoxic encephalopathy," which basically means a lack of oxygen has left the brain permanently damaged to the point where the patient suffers from total unawareness or coma.

Still others may be left in a "persistent vegetative state," like that of the famous life and death of Terry Schiavo, where the eyes are open and basic bodily functions continue, but the patient suffers from inability to interact and communicate with the outside world and perhaps complete unawareness.

Although in layperson terms, there may not seem to be much of a difference between brain death and these states, when it comes to leading end-of-life discussions or making end-of-life decisions, the difference is paramount.

Death on television or in the movies is that final instant, when the eyes close, the head slumps to the side and the heart ceases to beat. Death to the medical and scientific community might mean brain death, like Walter's, or the more common cardiac death when the heart ceases to beat and the brain dies afterwards.

But my experience with Walter, his family, and others like him makes me question all these different definitions, all these preconceived notions. The "time of death" is so arbitrary and subjective. Is it the moment the heart stops? When brain activity ceases? Is it neither? Is it both? Does death occur when awareness slips away, when consciousness or irreversible coma takes hold? Is it the moment when it's decided that the machines should be removed and a natural death allowed to occur?

There is no right answer, only interpretation.

The hardest part of explaining brain death, for me, is explaining to a family that they don't have a choice in whether we remove the ventilator and the machines. The words as they escape my lips sound so cruel: "You don't have a choice." By medical standards, and even legal standards, brain death is absolute in its finality. It's hard for me to find a way to say the words to these families, and no doubt even harder for them to hear and accept them.

The discussion and counselling is entirely different in the case of brain death than for the patient whose brain still lives while the body is dying. Those are the families who have to choose. Should we continue life support? Should we initiate dialysis? Should we give consent for yet another surgery? How much easier it would seem to them, I would think, to be spared the agony of having to decide just how far and how long they should continue to attempt to beat back death as it takes hold.

Unfortunately, this latter situation is the more common in a medical ICU. It's a few times per month that I meet a patient whom we formally diagnose as brain dead in the medical intensive care unit. More often, in the medical ICU, the situation occurs when the patient is less definitive, leaving a family to struggle with the decisions and choices, and how to move forward.

Once a patient arrives in the ICU and is stabilized, our first order of business is to figure out *who* will be making decisions and giving consents for medical treatments. It's ideal if the patient is still able to make his or her own decisions, but if not, we seek out either the power of attorney or next of kin. Sometimes the decision makers, or surrogates, know that they will have to make the choices. Sometimes, they don't. Sometimes they are prepared for this task, armed with the knowledge of what their loved one would want under such circumstances, and sometimes, they are less so.

Our surrogates become our voice when we cannot speak. They answer the 3 a.m. phone calls, to sign the papers and make the choices. Arming our surrogates with the information they need about our end-of-life wishes is of the utmost importance. The reality is that whether prepared or not, critical illness often arrives unannounced, and its consequences must be faced head on by those that we name as our decision makers and to speak on our behalf.

Discussion Questions

1. Why do you think it was hard for Walter's parents to understand to that he was dead, but still had vital signs on the monitor?

2. Once the doctors declared Walter brain dead, his parents had no end-of-life decisions to make, even though his heart was still beating. Why is this situation so unique?

3. How did you conceptualize the moment of death prior to reading Walter's story? How did his story change your perception, if at all?

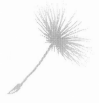

5

The Hospice Bride

Catching her breath as she approached Apartment 201, Rosemary rang the bell. While she waited, she looked admiringly at the handmade wreath on the door, clearly one of Barbara's creations, new in the week since Rosemary's last visit.

Rosemary's arm ached from holding up the gown she'd brought to the bride-to-be. To prevent the plastic from dragging on the ground, she shifted her weight and transferred it to the other arm just as Jeffrey opened the door.

"Close your eyes, Jeffrey! Don't look! Don't look!" Rosemary waved excitedly as he welcomed her into the apartment.

She could hear his fiancée, Barbara, calling from the living room. "Jeffrey, no peeking!"

Jeffrey shielded his eyes obediently and darted into the back bedroom as Rosemary hurried into the living room.

"Okay, Barbara, are you ready?" Rosemary's voice sang with excitement.

"Yes, yes, let me see it!" Barbara answered from her hospital bed. She now sat bolt upright, a feat she hadn't had the strength to accomplish just a few weeks earlier.

Rosemary swung the dress around so it was clearly within Barbara's view, and she peeled back the clear plastic that protected the fabric. Barbara shrieked with delight as her eyes took in the beadwork and lace.

"It's beautiful!" Barbara exclaimed. "It's just what I wanted! I can't believe it!"

"Well, believe it, honey, it's yours!" Rosemary said, hanging the dress up on the wall beside Barbara's bed. She was delighted at Barbara's reaction. In truth, the gown wasn't *exactly* what Barbara had asked for, but it was the closest thing the bridal shop had, and Barbara would never complain.

Rosemary mused, "Now, we'll have to figure out a way to get it on you . . ." She had been over it several times in her head already but was still quite anxious about how this would go. First, she was nervous about the measurements. Rosemary was a hospice worker, not a seamstress, and she had never measured anyone before, let alone someone who couldn't stand up. She'd done her best, but when she had first seen the dress, she was quite sure it was going to be too big. Then she worried about how she would get the gown on Barbara without calling Jeffrey in to help.

Barbara hadn't been out of bed in five years because of a cascade of serious illnesses. Just getting into a wedding gown was going to be a Herculean task. Yet Rosemary put the anxieties out of her mind, willing herself to be able to get the gown on Barbara without needing Jeffrey's help. They had been training for months for this day, and Barbara was in as good shape as she ever was going to be, so it was now or never.

Rosemary looked over at Barbara, whose smile had faded, her eyes still examining her wedding gown.

"It's too big," Barbara lamented. "I don't think it's going to fit."

"It's going to be fine—things always look bigger on the hanger. It's going to be fine." Rosemary hoped her voice sounded reassuring. "I have a plan. Don't worry."

Rosemary arranged a chair firmly against the wall near the bed and lowered the hospital bed as close to the ground as it would go. "All righty! Sit straight up and hold on to your tray, and we'll swing your legs over the side of the bed."

Barbara hesitated but followed Rosemary's direction, and she was able to get her body upright enough so Rosemary could easily slip off her silk nightgown in exchange for a soft, cream-colored camisole. Giggling and struggling, the two women contorted themselves until, finally, all the undergarments were where they should be and Barbara's weak legs dangled over the edge of her bed.

"Lean forward onto the chair to brace yourself," Rosemary instructed, laughing as they both struggled.

Barbara did as she was told, her gasps mixed with loud, deep laughter.

"You girls okay out there?" Jeffrey called from the back room.

"Yes! You stay put!" Rosemary commanded, feeling like a general leading her soldier to victory. "Barbara, don't move, just lean against the chair; it's braced against the wall."

As Barbara did so, Rosemary bolted to the opposite wall where the dress hung, uncomfortable leaving Barbara to fend for herself as she sat upright, away from the bed for the first time in ages. Barbara was giggling, but Rosemary knew that with just one mishap, Barbara could end up on the floor, which would be disastrous.

Rosemary ripped the dress off the hanger while lunging back toward Barbara to steady her. "Okay, here we go!"

Slowly and carefully, Rosemary slipped the gown over Barbara's head and pulled her arms through the sleeves one at a time. They shimmied and tugged for fifteen minutes until the gown fell into place, the skirt puffing out around the chair where Barbara sat.

"Now, the moment of truth," Rosemary prompted. "Lean forward and push with your legs like we practiced. You need to be up for only one second, and I'll pull the dress down over your hips."

Barbara furrowed her brow in concentration and stood, leaning hard on the chair. Rosemary yanked with all her might as the gown's skirt fell down over Barbara's hips into perfect position, and she slid the zipper to midway up her back.

"Okay! You can sit!" Rosemary shouted, louder than she needed to.

Barbara sat down, the look of victory in her eyes.

"Let's just get this zipped up, and we'll be in!" Rosemary held her breath as she pulled the zipper up to Barbara's shoulders.

"Does it fit?" Barbara asked. "Is it okay?"

Rosemary looked at Barbara from head to toe. Not only did it fit, but it was perfect.

The regional director for Innovative Hospice walked into his office just in time to hear his phone ring. He darted over to his desk and picked up the receiver without a chance to look at the caller ID.

"Hello?"

"Hi, Tim. It's Rosemary. Listen, there's a small problem with the invitations for the wedding."

He had to think for a moment. *Wedding? What wedding?* "Oh, for Barbara and Jeffrey!" he remembered, amused at his momentary memory lapse.

"Well, it's the invitations. Jeffrey's name is spelled wrong, and Barbara is really upset. It was our mistake, because we submitted the wrong spelling. They're gorgeous otherwise, but I was hoping that *Wish Upon a Wedding* might approve a reprint. It's not a catastrophe or anything, but years ago at Barbara's sister's wedding, Jeffrey's name was spelled wrong *and* he was put at a separate table from Barbara, and it caused a huge scene. Jeffrey's just sensitive to these things and Barbara is afraid he'll be upset—"

Tim interrupted. "I'm sure *Wish Upon a Wedding* will be fine with it, but you'll have to call the invitation printer to get an estimate."

"I already did: they're only going to charge one hundred fifty dollars," Rosemary said.

"Okay, I'll talk to Bob, the coordinator over there, and we'll see," Tim answered.

"Thanks, Tim. If he says no, I'll pay for it myself, but I've already picked up extra shifts so it would be hard—"

"We'll take care of it, either way," Tim assured her. "Just go ahead and order the reprint."

Rosemary squealed. "Thanks, Tim. I'll talk to you later."

Tim hung up the phone smiling wide. *Women*, he thought. *I just don't get it.*

Jeffrey had first met Barbara at a party when they were both seventeen years old. He'd never seen a prettier girl than Barbara, whose blonde hair was done neatly in a French twist with a tiny red flower perfectly placed on the side. She was seated at a picnic table next to her mother, with her hands folded neatly in her lap and her plate of food untouched in front of her. Barbara looked straight ahead, staring blankly into the garden by the side of the house. He saw a beautiful girl, gentle and kind, although, in actuality, he was seeing a person who didn't yet exist. What he didn't know was that she was heavily sedated with anti-psychotic medications and recovering from her last round of electric shock treatments.

He thought about her constantly and finally mustered up the courage to call Barbara's house two weeks later. They had spoken just briefly, and he had been so nervous that he had barely noticed Barbara's distant state and hadn't surmised that anything was wrong. Even on their first date, Jeffrey was so taken by Barbara's beauty and smitten by her shyness that he didn't think to question her monotone demeanor. It wasn't until Barbara's mother answered the telephone the following week and heard Jeffrey's intention to ask Barbara out on another date that he realized something wasn't quite right. Instead of putting Barbara on the telephone, her mother responded swiftly and angrily.

"Do not call here again," she said, leaving Jeffrey's mouth gaping as he listened to the dial tone.

Confused and frightened that he had done something dreadfully wrong, Jeffrey obeyed Barbara's mother's wishes and didn't try to call again, although he was heartbroken. Things started to make sense a few weeks later when he learned that Barbara had been taken to Burton Hospital, the local psychiatric ward, and a large "For Rent" sign appeared on the front of Barbara's family home.

Eighteen years passed, and Barbara was admitted to the psychiatric ward more than thirty more times. Ever since she was a little girl, Barbara's parents had moved to a new rental home or apartment each time she was released from hospital; they lived in a constant state of "damage control," refusing to acknowledge Barbara's illness to the outside world and keeping the depression, paranoia, and shock therapy a family secret. For Barbara, her teens and twenties slipped away into a medication-induced haze.

When Barbara was twenty-seven, she met a man named Brian at one of her group counseling sessions. After a short relationship, Barbara gave birth to a daughter, Jacquelyn. But the relationship with Brian didn't last, and soon after Jacquelyn's first birthday, Barbara moved back into a small apartment in Northeast Philadelphia with her mother, who helped her care for Jacquelyn. Barbara and her mother lived on a meager income, and Barbara's mother spent all the money they had playing Bingo. As a result of the dire social circumstances she faced, Barbara was continuously in and out of psychiatric hospitals, feeling withdrawn, distrusting, and neglected.

Her sole social support was her only friend from school, Janet.

Fatefully, Janet's brother was Barbara's old beau, Jeffrey, who had just returned from service abroad and had moved into Janet's apartment. He hadn't much in the way of formal education, so finding a job was a challenge, and he was feeling down. Janet invited Jeffrey to breakfast with Barbara and Jacquelyn in hopes that an outing would lift everyone's spirits.

When he arrived to the diner, Jeffrey was stunned to find the beautiful young girl he had once been so infatuated with sitting just a few steps away.

"Another Budweiser," Jeffrey said to the bartender, who nodded in response.

Jeffrey was sitting at a local bar trying to muster up the courage to go to the payphone in the corner.

"Just do it!" said another patron at the bar who had been witnessing Jeffrey's struggle for the last hour.

Jeffrey was anxious. He had met Barbara twice for breakfast with his sister, but he still wasn't sure how Barbara would respond if he asked her out for a second date, just the two of them, a full eighteen years after their first date.

"Okay, I'll try again," Jeffrey said, standing up from his bar stool. He dug into his pocket for more coins. This time, he was determined *not* to hang up when she answered.

Jeffrey finished off his second beer and headed boldly to the wall, feeling the eyes of the bartender and bar patron following him.

"Hello," a young voice answered.

"Hi, Jacquelyn," Jeffrey said, recognizing the little girl's voice. "Is your mom there?"

A few moments later, Barbara was on the other end of the telephone.

"Uh, hi, Barbara. This is Jeffrey. Jeffrey Stone. I, uh, was wondering . . ." He trailed off but quickly regained his composure, "My niece is getting married in a month. Would you like to go with me as my guest?"

When she answered yes, Jeffrey threw his arms up in the air in victory, sparking applause from the bartender and patron. He had a date with the girl with the red flower in her hair, and his grin didn't fade for the next ten years.

By age forty-five, Barbara's physical state had deteriorated. She had developed spinal stenosis, a painful condition that caused severe back pain. She underwent three back surgeries, none of which alleviated the pain and deformities she had developed. With each hospitalization and surgery, Jeffrey spent the night by her bedside. Since Barbara was still living in a two-bedroom apartment with her mother and her daughter, Jeffrey actually cherished the time at the hospital when he could stay with her. Although Barbara continued to need medical hospitalization, her psychiatric hospitalizations became fewer and farther between. Jeffrey's companionship and love brought pure happiness to Barbara, and slowly but surely she began to emerge from the darkness she had lived in her entire life. Like a butterfly, Barbara was coming out of her cocoon, fully becoming the person Jeffrey had imagined her to be so many years ago.

When Jacquelyn turned twenty-three, she got her first job working as an aide in the local hospital. Barbara was unable to work because of her back problems, and she collected disability insurance. After Barbara's mother died, things got even harder. Their financial situation was deteriorating, and Barbara's needs were worsening. Barbara needed help bathing, standing, and dressing, and it was becoming too much for Jacquelyn to handle on her own. As if it couldn't get worse, Barbara suffered a stroke, leaving her incredibly weak on her right side, and Barbara was right-handed. She was in the hospital for weeks, including the rehabilitation center, and Jeffrey helped Barbara with every step. A few days before she was finally ready to go home, Jacquelyn told her mother she was placing her in a nursing home since she couldn't keep up her job and care for Barbara in the way that she needed.

Jeffrey, of course, would hear nothing of it. Now with an apartment of his own, Jeffrey insisted that Barbara return home with him. He gave up his bedroom and created a makeshift bedroom for himself in the living room, sleeping on the sofa. For Jeffrey, it was a small price to pay in order to keep Barbara from being sent to a nursing home.

"You can't take care of her, either," Barbara's daughter erupted.

"I can and I will," Jeffrey insisted.

"You don't have enough space and certainly not enough money. She'll be better cared for in a facility. I'm not doing this to be cruel, Jeffrey, I'm doing this because its what's best for my mom," Jacquelyn sobbed. Her nerves were shot, and she felt like she was forty-three rather than twenty-three. She was tired, angry, and sick of all the illness in her life. She needed to get away from it, and she needed to be on her own.

After Jeffrey took Barbara home, the visits from Jacquelyn became fewer and fewer. Eventually, she stopped visiting at all.

Cancer struck next. Barbara had been suffering from nausea and stomach pains, and the doctors diagnosed her lymphoma, a form of blood cancer similar to leukemia. By this time, Barbara was fifty-five and almost completely bed-ridden because of the back injuries and stroke. In a whirlwind month, the doctors initiated chemotherapy in hopes that it would reduce the progression of the cancer. But after just six months of therapy and countless nights of intolerable nausea and yet another admission to the hospital, Barbara had had enough.

"It's possible this next round will be more effective," Dr. Ricardo told her, pulling up a chair alongside Barbara's hospital bed.

"I don't think so," answered Barbara, "and I'm not willing to deal with this nausea anymore. I'm tired, and I don't like the way it makes me feel. I want to go home with Jeffrey."

Dr. Ricardo looked into Barbara's eyes and saw a woman suffering. A glance over to Jeffrey revealed her boyfriend's pain as well.

"If you want to stop treatment and consider a palliative route, like hospice, I will certainly support your decision," he said. "You don't have to continue the chemotherapy, especially since it doesn't seem to be helping very much." It was almost as if he was convincing himself.

"I'll bring you home, Barbara. Your room is waiting for you, and maybe you'll feel better once you're home," Jeffrey said, his voice firm, steady, and resolute.

"All right, we have to do a lot of things first, though," Dr. Ricardo said. He was feeling anxious about this new turn of events. He wasn't sure that Barbara and Jeffrey truly knew the impact of what they were saying. If Barbara left the hospital, she would certainly die.

So he asked her, "Do you understand what this decision means, Barbara?"

"Doctor, I'm not afraid of dying. If the cancer spreads, it spreads. I know what hospice is and that the end is probably near. But what you have to understand is that for once in my life . . ." her voice trailed off.

"We're happy," Jeffrey finished. "And having her in and out of the hospital all the time, always vomiting and uncomfortable, is just taking away from our happiness."

Barbara nodded. Dr. Ricardo was amazed at how neither one of them was tearful or even hesitant with their words. Barbara was so vulnerable, so weak and emotionally challenged in so many ways, but what he saw in her eyes was anything but weakness.

"All right. If you and your husband agree, I'll call our palliative care team for you," Dr. Ricardo said. "We are going to try to help you get home."

Jeffrey and Barbara smirked at each other, and Dr. Ricardo's confused look prompted Jeffrey to explain.

"We're not actually married," Jeffrey said.

"But we may as well be," Barbara answered quickly.

"They told us we couldn't get married or we'll lose her health insurance," Jeffrey lamented.

Dr. Ricardo looked puzzled. "Well, I recommend then that you get a legal power of attorney signed, Barbara, if you want Jeffrey to be able to make decisions for you. Otherwise, it will default to your daughter if you ever become unable to make decisions on your own."

"How do I do that?" Barbara asked.

"Luckily, here in Pennsylvania it's just a simple form. We have them in the nurses' station, and I'll have Dotti bring one for you to fill out. You'll just need two witnesses to sign and that's it, " Dr. Ricardo answered.

"Hey, honey, we'll really be legal then!" Jeffrey said enthusiastically, "even if we aren't *really* married."

Dr. Ricardo just laughed. Jeffrey and Barbara seemed like teenagers, bonded by hardships and an innocent hopefulness. "You two are like two little lovebirds. I don't know the details of how getting married will affect your health benefits, but if there's any way around it, you ought to try and find it."

The next day, Jeffrey noticed Barbara was beginning to sweat. She had been running a low-grade temperature but had otherwise been doing well. Since they had finished the power of attorney form, Barbara had been upbeat although somewhat emotional. It may not have been a marriage certificate, but to Barbara, it felt just as good. Jeffrey had committed to taking care of Barbara, and loving her, to the very end. Before they signed the form, they symbolically wrote and recited vows, with two of Jeffrey's friends signing as the witnesses.

The ceremony had invigorated Barbara, and for once in her life, everything was perfect, her eyes beaming and her heart light. But the sweat on Barbara's forehead was beading and Jeffrey noticed the look on her face was changing.

"Are you okay?" he asked, feeling her forehead with the back of his hand.

Barbara just mumbled.

"I'll get you a washcloth for your forehead, honey," Jeffrey said soothingly. "I'll be right back."

Jeffrey knew where to go since he had been to the linen rack many times in the last few weeks to get Barbara fresh pillowcases, towels, and sheets. On his way, he saw Barbara's nurse, Dotti, and asked her to check on Barbara.

They soon learned that Barbara had more than a fever, she had sepsis, a severe inflammatory response to some sort of infection, which in Barbara's case, was a urinary tract infection. When Dr. Ricardo learned of the situation from the nurse, he came immediately to speak with Jeffrey.

"This is a difficult situation," Dr. Ricardo began gently. "You see, the infection that Barbara has goes beyond just a typical urinary infection. Since her body is weakened from the chemotherapy it can't fight the infection as effectively, and so it has caused her to have what we call sepsis, and I'm concerned that without aggressive treatment in the intensive care unit with antibiotics and possibly large neck IVs called central lines, she might not get well enough to ever make it home, which was our goal."

"I want to bring her back home with me," Jeffrey resolved. "She'll come out of this and then I can bring her home."

Dr. Ricardo pressed his lips together in thought. *Is this a reasonable goal in this situation?* he thought to himself. Certainly, sepsis was a reversible condition, something that could be treated, and if she responded, she might return to her normal status. But, if the infection didn't respond or it spread, and Jeffrey wanted full aggressive measures, Barbara would likely end up on a ventilator with little chance of making it home and would have gone through an extraordinary number of aggressive treatments in the process. Since Barbara had already made clear that she wanted to pursue a palliative treatment plan and not a curative one, Dr. Ricardo wanted to make sure Jeffrey understood what he was getting into.

"If we move her to the intensive care unit, she'll require a central line, aggressive hydration, a urine catheter called a Foley, and a lot of blood tests. I think there is a chance she'll respond, so I'm going to leave it up to you, Jeffrey. If you want to try and fight this sepsis so that we can get her home, we'll move her to the unit immediately," Dr. Ricardo said.

"Definitely," Jeffrey said.

After two weeks in the ICU, Barbara's situation had gotten worse instead of better. Her kidneys weren't working well, and she was in a constant delirious state. The ICU doctors told Jeffrey they were not hopeful that she would recover and recommended that he consider calling Barbara's daughter, since it was unlikely that Barbara would survive through the night. Since Barbara had been clear earlier that she did not want to be on life support, the doctors explained that they had done all they could and that Barbara's situation was so critical that if life support wasn't initiated, she would pass away.

Barbara had clearly told Jeffrey that she would rather pass away without life support than die hooked up to machines, and so Jeffrey picked up the phone to call Jacquelyn.

Despite the strained relationship, Jacquelyn came immediately to the hospital and spent hours weeping at Barbara's bedside. Jeffrey gave

Jacquelyn privacy and time alone with her mother, but even from outside the room he could hear her sobs in between the words *I'm so sorry.*

To everyone's surprise, Barbara didn't die. She remained unconscious, and the prolongation of her ICU course was distressing to everyone. This was a woman who had opted for palliative care just days before she had developed sepsis and yet they continued her care in the ICU. Barbara managed to survive even without the ventilator, and it was clear that if her heart were to stop, Jeffrey's choice would be not to have the doctors perform CPR. Yet the fact that Barbara was living on the edge of death, sustained by a feeding tube and medications to keep her blood pressure elevated seemed inconsistent with her wishes. When the doctors asked Jeffrey if it was time to stop and shut off the blood pressure medications and tube feeds, he resolutely said no.

"I want her fed," he said, "and I want the medications. I know she didn't want to treat her cancer, but if she has a chance to clear this infection, then I want to give her the chance. She's hung on longer than we expected already."

After a few more days, even Jacquelyn began to question whether it was time to let go and shut of the nutrition and blood pressure medications, although the decision was up to Jeffrey since he was the power of attorney.

But then, something miraculous happened. Barbara opened her eyes.

Four weeks later, Jeffrey opened the door and saw a middle-aged woman in nursing scrubs standing in front of him, smiling.

"Hello, I'm Rosemary," she said.

"Jeffrey."

They shook hands. Rosemary noticed Jeffrey's eyes were red and swollen. He had clearly been crying just moments before.

"May I come in?" she asked.

"Of course," Jeffrey fumbled as he opened the door wider and offered Rosemary something to drink.

"I'm just fine, thank you," she said peering around the apartment. It was drab with very little furniture and practically no decorations except a few small picture frames with pictures of Jeffrey and a woman who Rosemary presumed to be Barbara.

"She's right over here," Jeffrey said.

Rosemary peered into the living room where Jeffrey had gestured. There she first laid eyes on Barbara, her hair graying and frazzled, wearing a set of floral pajamas. Jeffrey had placed a bouquet of lilies, Barbara's favorite flower, by her bedside table, and a bed tray was cluttered with pill bottles and a barely eaten sandwich.

Rosemary had read Barbara's chart and was anxious about meeting the woman: the electric shocks, the numerous psychiatric medications, the cancer, the chemotherapy, the sexual abuse . . . Rosemary had no idea what sort of situation she was walking into.

A hospice nurse with more than eight years of experience, Rosemary loved her job. Twelve years prior to joining Innovative Hospice, she had worked as a surgical ICU nurse until her colleagues convinced her that she was missing her calling. In the surgical ICU, Rosemary was known as the go-to person for helping to comfort families struggling with end-of-life decisions. Rosemary had a gift for helping them come to terms with the difficult decision of removing their loved one from the ventilator, and she was the most skilled in providing comfort to the patients and their families in the setting of the ICU.

"You should become a hospice nurse," her co-workers would say over and over, until one day, she did.

Now, eight years later, she had never looked back.

"Hello, Barbara. I'm Rosemary," she greeted, cautious as she approached Barbara's bed.

"Hello." Barbara was weak from her bout with sepsis but had recovered enough at the hospital that finally, with Innovative Hospices' help, she had been able to come home. Although she had been lingering near death for weeks, the day Barbara opened her eyes, things had begun to take a turn for the better. Jeffrey had sat by her bedside each night, longing to hear Barbara speak or answer when he called her name. He had called the funeral home and a priest had come to read Barbara her last rites. The traumatic effect from that experience was not lost on Rosemary, and she knew that not only would she need to focus on providing supportive care for Barbara's physical symptoms and needs, but for her and Jeffrey's emotional needs as well.

Rosemary moved the chair from the foot of the bed and dragged it up next to Barbara's side.

"So," she said. "Where should we start?"

Barbara just shrugged.

"It must feel really good to be home," Rosemary nudged.

Nodding, Barbara answered, "Yes, I'm really happy to be back in my apartment where Jeffrey and I can sit together without people running in and out."

"Yeah, the hospital can be a really restless place," Rosemary agreed.

"It's too much commotion and noise," Barbara added.

"Well, I'm glad we were able to get you back home. For awhile there, we weren't sure you were going to make it," Rosemary said the words cautiously, hoping to catch a glimmer of Barbara's feelings about all that had happened.

"I'm right where I want to be," she said.

"So staying out of the hospital is a priority for you?"

"Oh, yes!" Barbara said, speaking with an energy in her words that wasn't there before.

"Well, part of my job is to make sure you stay here, happy and at home."

"That sounds good," Barbara said, smiling.

"Let me ask you this, Barbara: right now, what is most distressing to you?" Rosemary asked, purposefully leaving the question up for interpretation.

"I don't know," Barbara said slowly, "I wish I had more energy. I get tired really easily. It's hard to keep my eyes open sometimes."

"That's completely understandable, considering what you've been through. I wonder if you take any medications that are making you sleepy," Rosemary thought out loud, "do you have your discharge paperwork from the hospital?"

"Jeffrey would have it if we do," Barbara said.

Apparently, Jeffrey had been listening in from the kitchen since he came into the living room with the paperwork and handed it to Rosemary.

"Here you go," Jeffrey said, adding "I have all Barbara's papers in a file, organized by date."

"That's great," Rosemary encouraged, "it'll be really helpful to take a look through her medical records so I can be sure we're addressing all her needs."

As she spoke, Rosemary's eyes reviewed the discharge paperwork. Barbara was taking a lot of medications, but she didn't notice any that would be overly sedating. Her pain medications were at a pretty low dose.

"It looks like you're taking some pain medications which might decrease your energy level, but I don't see anything else glaring out at me," Rosemary said to Barbara and Jeffrey. "You still have a few days left on your antibiotics from the hospital, so maybe it's just a matter of letting your body recover. Hopefully the antibiotics will help eradicate any remaining infection and make you feel a little better."

"I've been on the same dose of pain medications for a long time," Barbara said. "Sometimes they make me tired, but not like this."

"Well, we'll keep an eye on your energy level over the next week or so and see what we can do," Rosemary said, still reading the paperwork Jeffrey had provided. Her job was to manage the medications from here on out, and she reviewed the list with a fresh eye, being that this was the first time she had ever met Barbara. Barbara was on antibiotics, pain medications, breathing treatments for shortness of breath, vitamins, and a few blood pressure medications.

"Do you have all these medications here?" Rosemary asked.

Jeffrey nodded. "Yeah, I picked them all up yesterday."

"Okay, good. It looks like you have almost everything you need. We can add some nausea medication, just in case," Rosemary said. "Sometimes the antibiotics can make your stomach a little upset."

"Yeah, I do have a little nausea," Barbara admitted.

Something about Barbara's medication list bothered Rosemary, and it took her awhile to figure out exactly what was wrong.

"Do you take any psychiatric medications?" Rosemary asked. She was shocked when she realized that there were none on the list. From everything she had heard about Barbara's mental illness and history, she thought for sure she should some psychiatric medications ordered.

"Most of them were stopped a few years ago. Since Barbara moved in with me, she hasn't been in a mental hospital at all," Jeffrey said proudly, "They started taking her medications away one by one because she was getting so much better. The only one left was a depression medicine which they stopped while she was in the ICU because they said it might interact with other medications she was on."

Rosemary nodded. She knew what medication Jeffrey was talking about because she remembered reading about the decision to stop it in the ICU chart. She wondered if Barbara's energy problem had an element of depression contributing to it. It was impressive that this woman, Barbara, had such a clear psychiatric turnaround after moving in with Jeffrey, making Rosemary smile to herself about the healing power of companionship and love.

"Our hospice doctor, Dr. Stocker, is going to come to see you tomorrow," Rosemary said, "and I'll see if he wants to add back your depression medication. Maybe it'll help your energy level."

"Okay," Barbara said, looking at Jeffrey, who shrugged at her in return, seemingly able to read her mind.

"I thought hospice got rid of most medications," Jeffrey inquired, clearly on Barbara's behalf.

"Oh, no! That's not necessarily true. We provide medications to help you feel well, whether they are antibiotics, depression medications, blood pressure medications . . . whatever you need to keep you from having unpleasant symptoms," Rosemary said with a smile. She was used to common misconceptions about hospice.

"I'll talk to the doctor later today, and he'll help out with whatever you need," Rosemary said. "In the meantime, I'll make sure we have all the supplies we need."

She reviewed the list of supplies that Innovative Hospice had ordered for Jeffrey and Barbara, made sure they had arrived, and checked that Jeffrey knew how to use the equipment, particularly the oxygen tank and tubing. She took the opportunity to evaluate Barbara's physical state and her home environment as well so she could write up her full nursing assessment and give her daily report to the physician. For Rosemary's first several sessions she focused on showing Jeffrey and Barbara how to use the medical equipment hospice had provided: the specialty hospital bed, the oxygen delivery system, the trapeze "pull-up" bar installed over the bed and the "pillow-seat" wheelchair. She gave them tips on how to maneuver and arrange the apartment to make it easiest for Barbara to wash, get to the bathroom and enjoy her own home.

But over time, it was more than just "stuff" that hospice was providing for Barbara and Jeffrey. In a home that once had very few visitors, suddenly, Jeffrey and Barbara found they had company almost every day. Dr. Stocker came once a month. Their personal social worker, Ebony, came weekly. The home health aide came five times a week to help with bathing and light housework and Rosemary, of course, came twice a week. From a life of being sheltered from others and living in shadows, Barbara found herself to be the center of attention and the recipient of more compassion than she had ever imagined. Although she couldn't go outside to enjoy the sunlight, she had new light from the people around her.

Within just a few months after being so close to death, Barbara had recovered much of her strength and was thriving both physically and mentally. Jeffrey was especially surprised to see how much Barbara she had perked up, and that eventually his worries shifted from her physical health and her symptoms to keeping her mind busy and content. With Rosemary's help, he set up an art station next to Barbara's hospital bed so that she could draw and work on , scrapbooks and crafts when she was feeling well. The tasks kept Barbara active, and Jeffrey hung each completed project proudly on the wall until their apartment, once barren and empty, came alive with color.

As Rosemary and Barbara were getting to know each other, Barbara began opening up about her tumultuous past, and Rosemary found herself leaving her visits until the end of her day so she could stay longer than the allotted hour. Their time together changed from a formal patient-nurse relationship to one reminiscent of old friends.

One afternoon when they were watching TV together, Barbara's cell phone rang in the kitchen, and she asked Rosemary, "Can you get that for me?"

"Sure." Rosemary got herself up from an armchair near Barbara's bed.

"Look at that!" Barbara cooed at the television. They were watching a live red carpet event for an awards show.

"Oh my goodness, she's gorgeous!" Rosemary said, glancing over her shoulder as she headed towards the kitchen.

"Hello?" she answered and listened to the caller, the smile fading off her lips, "Hold on for a moment, please."

"Barbara, it's Jacquelyn," Rosemary said, setting her eyes on Barbara's face to gauge her reaction. Rosemary knew that Jacquelyn had visited Barbara only once since Barbara had come home from the hospital.

Barbara remained stoic and nodded, turning down the volume on the television.

After handing the phone to Barbara, Rosemary slipped quietly toward the bedroom and wandered to the back of the apartment in an attempt to give Barbara some privacy, but by the time she reached the bedroom, Barbara called her back to the living room.

"Everything all right?" Rosemary said.

Barbara nodded. "Jacquelyn is coming to visit me tomorrow."

"How do you feel about that?" Rosemary asked cautiously.

"It'll be nice. I just hope Jeffrey doesn't get upset."

Rosemary said nothing, waiting for Barbara to continue.

"Jeffrey is really angry with Jacquelyn, and he has a hard time holding back his emotions," Barbara began. "I was in and out of the hospital for so long—my whole life—and once Jeffrey came back into my world, he never left me. He stayed every night but one, and that was because of a snowstorm."

Rosemary chuckled. "That's so sweet, Barbara. It must feel really good to have someone there for you like that."

Barbara nodded. "I never had anyone before. My mother kept me hidden and would call the doctors with the slightest problem. I was in the hospital more than I was home when I was younger, and ever since I started having back problems, then the stroke, then the lymphoma . . . it was a lot for Jacquelyn." She trailed off, tears welling in her eyes.

"You've had a really hard life, Barbara. A lot of really bad things have happened to you," Rosemary said. "I can't even imagine how sad you must be."

"No, see, that's the thing," Barbara said, her eyes cleared up immediately. "I'm so happy now. I'm not mad or sad. What has happened, happened. And I can't change it. Jeffrey has changed my life, made me happy, and I don't even care about all that stuff of the past."

Rosemary smiled. Although Barbara was bed-bound, she was stronger than anyone Rosemary had ever known.

"The problem," Barbara continued, "is that Jeffrey is angry with my family. He blames them, I think, for all the years we weren't together, and for all the years I was sick, the years he remembers but I can't. And he is still really mad at Jacquelyn for not visiting me all that time and for when she wanted to put me in a nursing home," she said. "He still hasn't forgiven her."

"Have you?" Rosemary said softly.

Barbara looked at Rosemary with gentle eyes. "Of course."

"Settle down, everyone," Tim said over the chattering crowd. "Let's get started. We've only got two hours today."

Tim ran the weekly interdisciplinary team meetings at Innovative Hospice, and today they had a long agenda to cover. At each meeting, the nurses, social workers, physicians and chaplains came together over breakfast and coffee to discuss every patient on the hospice service. Tim passed the meeting agenda and documents that would be reviewed as the conversations around the conference room table trickled down to a whisper and eventually stopped completely.

"All right, we have forty-two patients on service this week, so we're going to tackle half this week and half next week. We also have a few policies to review and a few other administrative tidbits. So let's just jump right into our new admissions. Crystal, do you want to go first?"

Crystal, a hospice nurse like Rosemary, still chewing her bagel, nodded enthusiastically. She swallowed, shuffled a few papers and started her report on a new patient, Mr. Levinsky, who suffered from chronic obstructive pulmonary disease, called COPD for short. This condition, which is often, but not always, due to cigarette smoking, is also sometimes called emphysema. She told the group about him and his condition, and one of the doctors on Mr. Levinsky's team also expressed concern that Mrs. Levinsky needed some help, as she'd been ill herself recently, and bathing and dressing her husband was taxing for her. The chaplain on the team talked about what he'd observed during his visits at the home, and the group decided to increase the frequency of his visits to support Mrs. Levinsky in the care of her husband.

Next, another hospice nurse, Gladys, updated her colleagues on the status of an eighty-seven-year-old patient with Alzheimer's dementia. Mr. Jackson's main issue waswas nutrition, and she praised his social worker for his help in counseling the caregivers, Mr. Jackson's daughter and her family, on how to address this issue.

Others reviewed their cases, and the meeting continued until everyone had given their reports. Rosemary had spoken about Barbara's care, and since things were going so well, they hadn't had a lot to discuss. The doctor was going to visit Barbara next week and renew her medications, and all the rest of the care plan was unchanged.

When all the coffee was finished and there was nothing but crumbs on the bagel platter in the center of the table, Tim closed his notebook and moved to quickly handle the few remaining administrative items

"In the back of your packet, you'll see a memo from a nonprofit called *Wish Upon a Wedding*," Tim said. "They have a great program where they put on weddings for people suffering from a terminal disease. All the vendors donate everything: the cake, the dress, the makeup, the photographer, everything is done by professionals in the wedding industry who volunteer. The Philadelphia coordinator offered to do a wedding for one of our patients if we have any that would be appropriate."

Rosemary, whose mind had already moved on to the rest of her afternoon plans, snapped back into the meeting and sat bolt upright in her chair.

"Barbara and Jeffrey would be perfect!" she exclaimed, her heart beginning to beat faster in hopes that no one else would want to offer their patients. Why hadn't she thought of this sooner?

"Great, I'll forward you the email from the coordinator, then," Tim said. "Be sure everyone has signed the roster and thanks everyone for coming."

Rosemary sat back in her chair with ideas racing in her head. In an instant, the meeting ended, and all her colleagues were standing up and stretching their arms and legs, yet Rosemary found herself motionless in her chair. A wedding was what Barbara and Jeffrey had always dreamed of, and just like that, Rosemary thought, their dream could come true.

"Just tell them your story," Rosemary said, encouragingly. "They'll be blown away."

Barbara looked anxious. "Well, we'll see. I don't want to get my hopes up. Weddings are so expensive and Jeffrey and I don't have any money. Plus, I'm still not sure about the issue with my health insurance."

"I know, but we'll take it one step at a time. Let's just see if they can do it before we get ourselves crazy or too excited," Rosemary agreed. But she knew full well that she already had *her* hopes up probably higher than they should be, and that if they were accepted, they wouldn't have to pay a cent.

There was a knock on the door and Barbara and Rosemary's eyes locked, both with a flurry of excitement sparking between them.

"Here we go!" Rosemary said, her voice cracking from the excitement as Jeffrey emerged from the kitchen to open the door.

"Hello," Jeffrey greeted, "come in, come in!"

After the greetings and pleasantries abated, the two gentlemen from *Wish Upon a Wedding* sat down at the chairs Jeffrey and Rosemary had arranged at Barbara's bedside.

Barbara's smile was from ear to ear, and Rosemary noticed that Jeffrey was gripping his hands together with anxiety.

"This is going to be really informal," said the first man who had introduced himself as Larry. "Kevin and I are here to get an overview of your story and see if there is a good fit for you and *Wish Upon a Wedding*. I don't want you to think of it as an audition, though, all right?"

Barbara and Jeffrey nodded and Rosemary drifted to the back of the room, keeping her eyes firmly on Barbara to offer her silent support.

"So, let's start by telling me how you met," Larry said.

Jeffrey smiled, looked at Barbara and then at the men, and began.

Rosemary snuck brief glances at the notes Kevin was taking while Jeffrey spoke. She squinted to read as he wrote, but his handwriting was sloppy enough that she couldn't make out much of it. Then, about ten minutes into Jeffrey and Barbara's interview, Rosemary saw Kevin jot a quick note to Larry, which he underlined three times and then circled before tilting the pad so Larry could read it: "Does it get any more perfect than this?"

Two months later the wedding plans were in full swing. *Wish Upon a Wedding* had assigned Gloria, a professional wedding planner, to help coordinate Barbara and Jeffrey's wedding. Gloria was a young, enthusiastic woman, with short blonde hair and a face that could easily have graced the covers of glamour magazines. She wore fitted skirts and collared shirts to all her meetings with Barbara and Jeffrey, and she carried a briefcase filled with wedding vendor information, sample invitations, and photographs of cakes and all the other tools of her trade. Things were happening fast, and the team at Innovative Hospice was working furiously to make all the necessary medical arrangements to get Barbara out of her home and to the wedding venue. Rosemary was running to and fro, taking care of her other hospice patients and helping Barbara make wedding decisions on her lunch breaks and evenings.

"Too scripty," Barbara said, as Rosemary was going over the wedding invitation samples Gloria had left the day before. "I can barely read it!"

"How about this one?" Rosemary said, handing Barbara an invitation with a deep purple background, cream-colored lettering and a lavender ribbon that dangled off the corner.

Barbara smiled broadly.

"I like this one a lot!" Barbara exclaimed. "Do you?"

Rosemary nodded, "It's gorgeous."

"I can't believe this is happening," Barbara said, turning the invitation over in her fingers. "I never knew people like this existed! I mean, who would just offer to give Jeffrey and me a wedding for free?"

"There are lots of people in this world who do care," Rosemary said soothingly, "and you and Jeffrey deserve this."

"And you're sure that I'll still have health benefits?"

Rosemary giggled. "Yes, for the hundredth time, yes! The hospice doesn't care if you're married, and quite frankly, I'm not even sure where that idea came from. I promise you, you'll have everything you need. And you'll be Mrs. Jeffrey Stone on top of it!"

Rosemary knew that the social worker, Ebony, had done some investigation about the issue and hadn't found any barriers to Barbara and Jeffrey getting married. Barbara and Jeffrey relied heavily on Ebony's social work expertise. Whenever Barbara had any kind of medical paperwork or insurance issue, she'd show the documents to Ebony, who would explain them to Barbara and Jeffrey. With all the complexities, Barbara and Jeffrey were easily overwhelmed and Ebony had been a godsend for them in that regard.

"Ebony took care of everything," Rosemary reassured.

Tears welled up in Barbara's eyes. "I just still can't believe it. It's actually going to happen!"

"Well, I think this is a perfect invitation, don't you?" Rosemary said, refocusing Barbara on the task at hand. They had a lot to accomplish tonight. Gloria had deadlines for choosing the flowers and the invitations as well as selecting the menu. Although Barbara wanted to let Gloria choose whatever she thought was best, Rosemary knew that planning a wedding would keep Barbara's mind active and happy. It was the ultimate project.

"Will you be my maid of honor?" Barbara said suddenly as Rosemary was pulling out a booklet of flower bouquets.

"Huh?"

"I really want you to be my maid of honor," Barbara repeated.

Rosemary leaned down and hugged Barbara. "I would be so honored to, Barbara, but don't you think you should ask Jacquelyn?"

"I know, but you're the one who I really feel closest to. You're my closest friend and if it weren't for you, none of this would be happening."

"Well," Rosemary hesitated before answering. One of the hospice team's goals was to help Barbara, Jeffrey and Jacquelyn reconnect and strengthen their relationship. Both Rosemary and Ebony had spent hours with all three of them separately to help them deal with the issues of the past and to help them nurture healthy relationships moving forward. Since Barbara was, after all, on hospice, closure and relationship development was an important part of her overall care. Rosemary feared that by agreeing to be the maid of honor, she could potentially be interrupting all the progress Barbara and Jacquelyn had made in their relationship. Barbara had come to think of her hospice team as family, and Rosemary too felt a closeness and bond with Barbara unlike any other patient she had cared for. Part of Barbara's progress emotionally had been not only from her relationship with Jeffrey, but also with the connection she was forging slowly but surely with Jacquelyn.

"How about I be the one to push you down the aisle in your wheelchair?" Rosemary said, the idea coming suddenly to her.

Barbara looked disappointed for a moment, but then nodded in agreement.

"Okay, I think that's a good idea. But in my mind, Rosemary, you're my maid of honor," she answered. "Jeffrey thinks so, too."

Rosemary laughed. "Well, you're going to be the most amazing bride. I can't wait to push you down that aisle, and speaking of it, we should work on your exercises to get your strength up. It's going to be a long day for you, and we have to be ready!"

"Oh, believe me, Rose. I'll be ready!"

On the day of the wedding, the makeup artist arrived right on time as the wedding party assembled at Jeffrey and Barbara's apartment to help prepare the bride. Rosemary and Jacquelyn had worked together to dress Barbara, which made the task significantly easier than when Rosemary had done the fitting on her own. The ambulance was scheduled to arrive at 3 o'clock to take Barbara to the venue. Also going with her: Rosemary had ordered two oxygen tanks as backup and prepared an emergency medical toolbox, which she covered in a lavender satin to match the flowers and invitations. The video crew from *Wish Upon a Wedding* was recording the entire event, and they brought in movie lighting and backdrops to photograph Barbara, Rosemary and Jaquelyn being made up by the makeup artist. Jeffrey had already left to meet his family and groomsmen at the venue, and the apartment was buzzing with activity as Gloria fielded phone calls from the florist and caterers. Rosemary worried that all the excitement would wear Barbara out before the event even began.

"You feeling all right?" Rosemary asked in between photos.

"My face hurts from smiling," Barbara said. "I've never had so many photographs in my life."

"Well, you look great, and if it gets to be too much, just let me know and we'll take a break."

Ebony and Rosemary made eye contact. In all the excitement for the wedding, they hadn't anticipated such a whirlwind of activity to be around Barbara, and they silently shared their concern. Rosemary felt her stomach turn. Perhaps this was a bad idea after all. Maybe it was too much for Barbara. She was, after all, a terminally ill and physically weak woman.

Yet things moved along with Gloria keeping a close eye on the clock to ensure the makeup, photos and video didn't delay their arrival to the wedding hall.

"Time to go!" Gloria called over to Barbara, from across the apartment. "Can't be late!"

The paramedics and ambulance driver were seated in the kitchen, waiting for their cue. What a scene this must be for them, and how untypical this patient run must seem, Rosemary thought.

Ebony had already arranged for a motorized wheelchair to be delivered to the wedding hall, on rental for the day. The plan was to move

Barbara to the ambulance on a stretcher and transfer her to the wheelchair once they arrived at the hall. There wasn't much point in wasting her energy before the ceremony.

The paramedics sprung into action and whisked Barbara into the ambulance with seemingly little effort. Her wedding gown overflowed off the stretcher, so Rosemary and Jacquelyn carried the extra fabric to keep it from dragging on the ground. Gloria followed behind, chattering away on her cell phone. Once they approached the street where the ambulance was parked, Gloria snapped her phone closed and ran to the middle of the street to halt the oncoming traffic. Barbara, who hadn't been outside for many months, let alone with such a seemingly royal escort, was overwhelmed by all the commotion, and a look of joy, anxiety and happiness radiated from her. At first, passersby in the streets looked concerned upon seeing the paramedics lifting a bride into an ambulance, but on closer watch, seemed to understand what was happening, and raised their cell phones in the air to snap pictures like paparazzi, further cementing Barbara's role as queen for the day.

As soon as the sound of the wedding march began, Rosemary teared up. She was such a sucker for weddings. The moment was here, and before she could say a word of encouragement to Barbara, the double doors swung open, and they saw the aisle in front of them with the wedding guests flanked at either side.

Rosemary reached down to unlock the break on the wheelchair and began to push with some help from the motor that Barbara controlled. Her eyes scoured the hall, feeling overwhelmed at how many guests had turned out for the event. Not only had Jeffrey's entire family showed up, but she found Tim and the management team from Innovative Hospice in the back row as she pushed Barbara's chair forward into the room. As they ascended the aisle, she saw the hospice physicians, including Dr. Stocker. Further up, Ebony sat with a cluster of social workers and nurses who smiled and nodded as they met Rosemary's eyes.

Barbara's eyes were locked on Jeffrey, whose eyes locked right back on her. He wore a black tuxedo and a small red flower pinned to his lapel, the very same flower that he remembered from Barbara's hair at the picnic the day they had first met. She smiled when she saw the flower, remembering how silly she had been just days before. She had been annoyed at Jeffrey for insisting on a red flower rather than the lavender flower that matched the rest of the wedding colors. She leaned back in her wheelchair, feeling Rosemary's presence and support as she gripped the bouquet of lilies that rested in her lap.

Although the moment lasted only a few seconds, Barbara's trip down the aisle gave her a feeling of happiness that flooded her like no other moments in her life. The guests looked at Barbara and saw a beaming bride, not medical equipment, oxygen tanks or tubing. Instead, they saw the real-life fairytale.

"You did a wonderful job here," Tim said to Rosemary during the dinner reception.

"I didn't really do anything," Rosemary said modestly, "it was all Gloria and *Wish Upon a Wedding*. Everything went off without a hitch."

"I'm not talking about the wedding," Tim replied warmly. "I'm talking about Barbara's overall care."

Rosemary looked to her feet before looking back up at Tim.

"She's helped me just as much as I've helped her."

Tim tilted his head but said nothing.

"Before I met Barbara," Rosemary continued, "I was feeling so helpless. We get our hospice patients so late in the process. They come from the ICUs or so near death that there isn't a lot I can do to offer them support, other than treat their symptoms. We usually find ourselves working mostly on supporting the families, but with Barbara, I've gotten to know her as a person, not as a woman who is dying. And it's helped me do what I signed up for in this line of work."

Rosemary looked over to the table where the newly married couple sat. They were feasting on steak and crab, although the nurse inside Rosemary noticed that Barbara had barely touched her food.

"Well, it's been a wonderful day," Tim agreed. "Go enjoy it."

Rosemary looked at her watch. She and Ebony were seated in the atrium, enjoying a momentary break from the music. Rosemary listened as the song Barbara selected for the final song blared over the speakers.

"I'm beat," Rosemary said, resting her head on Ebony's shoulder.

"Me too," Ebony said. "Where are you parked?"

Rosemary didn't reply. Her stomach was up in her throat as she realized she had made a dreadful mistake.

"What's wrong?" Ebony said, sensing the change in Rosemary's demeanor.

Rosemary's mouth just gaped open.

"What?" Ebony insisted. "What's the matter?"

"We didn't book an ambulance home for Barbara," Rosemary said quietly.

Ebony opened her mouth, then closed it again. The realization hit the women like a brick wall.

"Maybe Gloria did?" Ebony squeaked hopefully.

"No. I'm certain she didn't," Rosemary lamented. "I knew that I was forgetting something!"

"It's all right. It's all right," Ebony started walking in small circles to offset the panic. "Just call the emergency hospice line and we'll set it up now."

"Oh, my gosh. I can't believe this," Rosemary dialed her phone furiously. "How could we be so stupid?"

"Well, this wedding went off way too perfectly. This little problem makes it a bona fide wedding, right? All weddings have catastrophes. This just happens to be an unusual problem." Ebony was speaking a mile a minute.

"I mean, who plans a wedding ambulance? It's just not something most people would think of. I dunno," she said sarcastically, "too late to rent a convertible?"

The ambulance arrived at 1 in the morning, and it was clear that Barbara was exhausted. In fact, Rosemary noticed that soon after the wedding cake had been cut, Barbara had dozed off in her wheelchair. The guests had left and Ebony, Rosemary, Jeffrey, and Barbara sat in the lobby of the hall waiting for the ambulance to arrive. Barbara's eyes were heavy but her heart and mind were light with joy, even as she slept. Jeffrey, too, was exhausted. The night had been incredibly emotional for him, filled with toasts, blessings and love.

"She's tuckered out," he noticed, yawning himself.

"The ambulance will be here soon," Ebony said. "Or it better be, because they're closing the hall down around us!"

No sooner had the words escaped her lips than the ambulance arrived, and two paramedics hopped out to pick up their patient.

"I'm so sorry about this," Rosemary greeted. "It's totally my fault that we forgot!"

"No problem at all," said the driver. "This is certainly a first for me, though!"

The paramedics pulled down the ambulance ramp and lifted Barbara out of her chair and onto the stretcher. As they loaded Barbara into the back, Jeffrey climbed in alongside her and collapsed on the bench that lined the wall of the ambulance, leaning his head against the back wall that was lined with oxygen masks. With a sigh of relief, Rosemary snapped one last photo of the wedding couple before the paramedics climbed in and pulled the door shut behind them.

"Don't worry," said the driver as he ensured the door was secure. "We came prepared."

Ebony shrugged at Rosemary as the driver disappeared around the side of the ambulance. He re-emerged carrying a cluster of oxygen masks tied along a length of rope, which he tied to the back door of the ambulance so that they dangled to the ground.

Ebony and Rosemary laughed out loud.

"It's perfect," Rosemary giggled.

"No, not yet," Ebony disagreed as she reached into her handbag. She plucked out her lipstick. "It's my favorite color and it's a shame to ruin it, but this simply won't do."

She popped the lid off the lipstick tube and scrawled "JUST MARRIED" on the back of the ambulance door.

"Now we can go!" the driver said with a smile. As he headed for the driver's seat Rosemary snapped one last photo of the ambulance pulling away to deliver the newlyweds home.

AFTERWORD

I interviewed Barbara and Jeffrey four months after their wedding. When I first arrived at their quaint apartment I knew very little about their story and was excited to hear more about the fairytale wedding my friends at Innovative Hospice had shared with me. I hadn't participated in a home visit since medical school, and I felt grateful that my role as a writer was allowing me to cross over the barrier from hospital to home and spend more time getting to know someone who is terminally ill outside the ICU where I usually see my patients. Still, I felt like an intruder as I stepped into the apartment, but Barbara and Jeffrey made me feel immediately at home.

Jeffrey had placed a chair at Barbara's bedside for me so that I could interview her. It looked strange to me, this chair in the middle of their living room, poised next to a hospital bed where Barbara laid amidst crafts, flowers, and other small treasures.

I had a list of questions in my head. *How did Barbara decide to enroll into hospice? Was she happy with her choice? What sorts of benefits and medications did Innovative Hospice provide her with? Was it expensive? What were Rosemary's visits like? What did the hospice clinicians actually do when they were visiting in the home?* The list was endless, and I had only a few precious hours to listen and learn.

At the time, I wasn't sure how ill Barbara was, since I didn't know much about her medical history then, but Barbara looked nothing like a woman on hospice to me. In fact, she looked like, well, a woman in bed. She wore a floral blouse. Her hair was done with some curls pinned up on the back of her head, and she wore just enough makeup to flush her face with color. Her oxygen tubing sat under her nose and around her neck. She was smiling. Death was not in the room.

When the conversation turned to hospice and its role in their lives, both Jeffrey and Barbara lit up with joy, and the conversation turned immediately to Rosemary.

"With Rosemary," Barbara smiled, "we talk about everything *except* for illness. We talk about life, about our families, about the things I do here. We don't talk about death or dying."

"You can't run from it, you have to face it," Jeffrey told me when I asked him about how he felt when Barbara had decided to enroll on hospice, knowing that patients are eligible for hospice if their doctors suspect they have less than six months to live. Instead of seeing hospice as the way in which Barbara would die, he instead spoke of how hospice was the way in which she would live. He spoke about the years when Barbara's family hid her psychiatric illness from public view, lived in denial and about the impact those years had on Barbara's psyche.

"It broke her confidence," he told me, "all those years. You can't hide, you have to move forward." As he talked, he pointed to the art and crafts that Barbara had created in the time she was receiving hospice care. He showed me drawings and photos, and although I tried to get him to talk about how he felt about his wife's impending death, he spoke only about the way in which she was living. When Barbara first enrolled in hospice care, she was near death, once again cocooned inside an illness, frequently hospitalized. However, once the needles, the IVs and the chemotherapy had been stopped, Barbara re-emerged.

"I never thought it would be like this," Barbara tells me. "It's been a blessing."

"But aren't you concerned that your cancer may have spread?" I asked.

"I'm not afraid of dying," she answered. "I don't know if I my cancer has spread. I don't fear that. I'm not scared. I know that, in all probability, it has spread somewhere. I do know that. But I'm still not afraid. I just don't care. I'm home with Jeffrey, and these days have been wonderful. And now we're even married. The cancer was a part of my life, and it's over with. If it spreads, it just is. There's nothing I can do about it." She paused. "Well, there is, but I simply choose not to. And that's okay."

Misperceptions about hospice run rampant, and Barbara and Jeffrey's story helped me to understand that hospice does so much more than to just help patients "die well." The hospice team literally transformed Barbara and Jeffrey's life and empowered them to think beyond the words *terminal disease*. Hospice, which is a fully covered Medicare benefit, provides its patients with medical, spiritual, and social services filling needs that many doctors overlook. After reading dozens of brochures from countless hospice agencies, including lists of services and benefits, it was after my time with Barbara and Jeffrey that the information in the brochures fell into context. Hospice goes beyond symptom management and pain control by offering not only medical care but also companionship, a caring team, counseling, home aides, spiritual guidance, and bereavement support after the patient has passed on.

Tragically, most patients who enroll in hospice care receive services for less than two weeks before they die. Usually, this is due to the fact that physicians refer patients to hospice much too late in their disease or because patients and families may resist the perception of giving up commonly associated with hospice care. Jeffrey and Barbara's experience exemplifies the tremendous opportunities in having hospice care for an extended period of time, instead only days or weeks before death. The hospice team that changed their lives as Rosemary gained control and alleviated most of Barbara's symptoms, as Ebony researched the implications of a legal marriage for Barbara and Jeffrey and even enabling them to be granted the wedding of their dreams, would not have been able to perform these miracles in only a few weeks. Barbara and Jeffrey had no problems with their medical benefits after their marriage and Barbara continues to take medications for pain, nausea, and shortness of breath. Some research studies suggest that patients who enroll in hospice care actually live longer than those with similar disease severity who opt for aggressive care. Certainly, in a lot of ways, they live better. Barbara has lived on hospice for almost two years, and continues to thrive.

During our interview, Barbara and Jeffrey were courageous in telling me and allowing me to write the truth about Barbara's life, including the unpleasantries behind Barbara's amazing journey.

"Well," Jeffrey said when I asked him to tell me his side of the tale, "it depends if you want to hear the real story or the fairy tale." But what he didn't realize was that they were one and the same.

Discussion Questions

1. After reading Barbara's story, did your perceptions of hospice care and its benefits change and if so, how?

2. There are many misconceptions about hospice care. Think about and discuss how Barbara's experience is contrary to the following misconceptions:

    a. Hospice care means stopping all medical therapies and medications.
    b. Being on hospice means you're giving up.
    c. People who enroll on hospice always die within a short period of time.
    d. Hospice is very expensive.

3. Some say hospice is a way to die, but Barbara says that it is instead a way to live. How do you feel about the idea of hospice care?

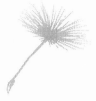

6

A Peaceful Passing

It all started with a sneeze. Sitting on her porch, comforted by her rocking chair, Victoria sneezed three times in rapid fire. She looked over at the blossoms dangling from a tree nearby. The allergies were back, and she'd better go inside and lie down. The same thing had happened yesterday, and she didn't want her throat to close up like that again. Victoria had lived in her house for a long time and always enjoyed a quiet afternoon on the porch, but over the last few months, she couldn't stay out for very long before her allergies started to act up. *I'm too old for this,* she thought.

She didn't know how true a statement that was. Seventy-nine-year-old women don't suddenly develop new allergies.

Victoria was a strong woman, a healthy woman who didn't even fathom that there could be anything else wrong. Once inside her house, she shooed the cat off the sofa and laid down for a quick nap. Victoria kept a tidy home, and things were always in their correct place. There was not a speck of dust to be found, and the only "clutter" you could find rested on her mantle, which teamed with ornately framed photographs of her children and grandchildren. There were eight frames in all and each frame contained a portrait of her respective daughters and sons with their children. There were forty smiling faces peering out from their portraits, looking over her as she slept.

But after a few hours, her allergies worsened despite the fact that she had been indoors for quite some time. The breathlessness was increasing, and she didn't feel like herself. She lifted the phone and called 911 because she needed some strong allergy medicine and she needed it soon. She felt a little silly, bringing in paramedics for an old lady with an allergy attack, but she didn't know what else to do. After the call, she went upstairs to put on her new blouse and slacks. She tied the laces on her black leather shoes and went downstairs to wait for the paramedics to arrive. She was surprised at how exhausted she was just after changing her clothes and the flight of stairs, but she felt better once she was back on the sofa. She picked up her knitting to distract herself while she sat in her quiet house. Gosh, she hated hospitals—all the noise and all the fuss. Her cat purred beside her, and Victoria made a mental note to pick up some cat food on her way back home.

The result of the x-ray was back about thirty minutes later. The doctor was young and handsome, but Victoria couldn't pronounce his name. All she knew was that he had just told her she had cancer.

Victoria's daughter, Lana was driving to the hospital a few hours later. Victoria had sounded pretty calm on the phone, so Lana knew that it wasn't that bad. Her mother had been suffering from terrible allergies, and she was certain that she would learn that her mom had developed pneumonia. She just hoped it wasn't too debilitating. Victoria was so independent, and Lana knew she wouldn't take well to being sick. Mom had the tendency to try and do more than she could handle, so Lana would have to keep a close eye on her to make sure she didn't overextend herself. If Mom was sick, Lana knew it was going to be up to her to take care of her. Not that she minded, but it wasn't exactly part of her master plan. Work was getting busier just now, and she didn't need the added stress of trying to convince her Mom to go to doctors' appointments. Mom hated doctors and hospitals, so Lana would have to be vigilant to make sure she kept up with whatever medical care this illness required. Lana knew she'd have to take charge, and she would.

The nurse, who was anxiously awaiting the doctor's arrival, greeted Dr. Olson at the door and told her that Victoria seemed more short of breath over the last few hours and that she was now on the maximum amount of oxygen that her nasal tube could emit. Dr. Olson nodded and sat down at the nursing station with the chart, which was mercifully thin. She opened the chart and began to read. The story was pretty typical: a newly diagnosed colon cancer with spread to the lungs. The patient had presented with complaints of an "allergy attack." How bad could this shortness of breath really be then?

The oncologists were evaluating whether Victoria was a surgical candidate and if she would require chemotherapy. Dr. Olson couldn't really read the oncologist's handwriting, but it didn't matter. She was here to assess the patient's shortness of breath and see whether she needed to be moved to intensive care. Once she gathered the story from the chart, she headed to the room to meet Victoria.

Victoria was in the room at the end of the hall, the nicest one on the wing because it had a large window overlooking the picnic area. In a way, it seemed cruel, Dr. Olson thought, allowing the patients to see all the healthy people eating their lunches outside in the perfect weather while they were trapped in their hospital beds, although she knew that the light and the window in itself could be healing. She was thinking about the window when she walked in the room and found Victoria sitting in the chair beside her hospital bed.

With each breath, Victoria's neck muscles contracted violently and it took her two full syllables to say "hel"-gasp-"lo." This wasn't an allergy attack. This was a woman in severe respiratory distress. Dr. Olson surveyed the room. Victoria's vital signs were displayed on the monitor: heart rate was fast, breathing was fast, but her blood pressure was okay. The oxygen saturation was at 90 percent. That was bad. On full nasal oxygen she was *only* at 90 percent. Dr. Olson called for the nurse to get a non-rebreather mask, which is capable of delivering 100 percent oxygen. She felt her own heart rate start to rise as she contemplated where to start and what to do next.

And then, Dr. Olson was stopped dead in her tracks. It was Victoria's eyes. They were calm. They were so calm, despite the fact that she was breathing at a rate twice as fast as a normal person would breath. Suddenly and without warning, Dr. Olson felt calm, too. She was struck by the contagious serenity Victoria exuded and the lack of fear on her face. She sat on the bedside next to Victoria and introduced herself. With all the external chaos, Dr. Olson wanted to be certain that Victoria knew who she was and what her role was.

"I'm Dr. Olson, and I am one of the residents working in the intensive care unit tonight. Your doctors asked me to come evaluate you because you are having such a hard time breathing, so I'm here to see if I can help you."

Victoria nodded in understanding and managed a feeble smile at the young doctor.

Sitting down next to her, Dr. Olson listened as Victoria tried between gasps to tell her how her shortness of breath was getting worse and worse, that she felt like she was suffocating. The words were slow, and it was a great effort for Victoria to get them out, but Dr. Olson listened patiently, encouraging Victoria to take her time in telling her what she wanted her to know.

By the time she had finished, Victoria could barely complete a sentence, which made it clear that there wasn't much time before she would require a ventilator to stay alive. Dr. Olson needed to see the x-ray. She strongly suspected a cancer-related pleural effusion, fluid in the lung that can easily be removed. She stepped outside to the x-ray computer and pulled up the films. Here eyes widened at what she saw: no fluid, but it was like a tumor gun had been aimed at Victoria's lungs. Tumor "bullets" had lodged all over her lung fields. It was incredible, unlike anything she had ever seen. Worst of all, one of the many tumors obstructed a bronchus.

This was far from an easy fix. This was a huge tumor that would kill Victoria, and it would kill her soon.

After Dr. Olson got over her shock, she paged Dr. Fred Bernstein, the intensive care fellow and her boss that night, to update him about her evaluation of Victoria. She was eager to hear his suggestions about what she should do, as he had much more experience than she did.

"I think we need to intubate her now, Fred!" Dr. Olson had told him the whole story, trying to sound confident when in fact she had never made that decision on her own before. With that, Dr. Bernstein had hung up the phone, run up the three flights of stairs separating him from Dr. Olson, and arrived huffing.

The next five minutes set everything in motion. Dr. Olson reached Victoria's daughter, Lana, on her cell phone (amazingly, despite all her shortness of breath, Victoria was able to recall this number without hesitation) while Dr. Bernstein reviewed the chart. Lana said she was fifteen minutes away from the hospital, and that made both Dr. Olson and Fred heave a sigh of relief. They all knew that if they did end up putting Victoria on the ventilator, she would probably never come off. Ever. They wanted to hold off as long as possible to allow Lana to be able to speak to her mom before they induced the artificial coma she would require to keep her pain-free while on the ventilator. It would probably be the last time Lana ever spoke to her mother, and since she was that close to the hospital, it meant that they could wait.

An experienced nurse was in Victoria's room hooking up the non-rebreather oxygen mask. Karen had worked in the cancer ward for twenty-something years, and she knew what was about to happen. Luckily, her other four patients were all stable at the moment, so she could devote all her time to helping with the situation in Victoria's room. She was impatient, too, wondering what was taking the doctors so long. Why hadn't they called for a bed in the intensive care unit yet? Twenty minutes had gone by since the doc was there, and still no one had called in the transfer.

Karen had been trying all night to help Victoria breathe easier, but nothing had helped. They had done breathing treatments, increased the oxygen in the nasal mask, changed her positioning in the bed, but nothing had worked. That's when she had called the intern, who had called for the unit evaluation. It seemed like an awful long chain of command to her, but that was what a teaching hospital was all about. Call the interns first; they'll call their senior residents who will call the fellows who will call the attendings. She had worked at non-teaching hospitals before, but she actually preferred the teaching hospitals. More doctors around. True, they were younger and inexperienced, but they were right there, in-house.

The oxygen rushed into the mask with a whoosh once Karen flipped the switch. She stepped outside to Victoria's room to see what plan the two doctors had conjured. She met them standing just outside Victoria's doorway.

"When are you going to move her?"

"Not yet. We need to stabilize her first," answered Dr. Olson, sensing the panic in the nurse's voice.

"So, you're just going to wait for her to code?"

Dr. Olson was relieved when Dr. Bernstein answered for her. "She's okay for now. Let's give the non-rebreather a chance to get her oxygen up, and then we'll move her to the unit."

Karen spun on her heels and walked back into the room. She had to get this patient off the floor. They weren't equipped here to deal with the level of care she needed. The sooner they got her off the floor, the better. Victoria was getting worse by the minute, and the transfer process and paperwork was lengthy.

By now, other nurses were arriving to check out the scene, and Dr. Olson felt a strong sense of "us versus them." She could hear the words of the nurses standing around the floor: "She needs to go to the unit *now,*" and "You've got to be kidding. They haven't called in the bed yet?" Dr. Olson felt a lump in her throat. Maybe they were right, and they should move her immediately, but the thought of wheeling a patient across the hospital while she was in distress didn't sit right with Dr. Olson. Just get the oxygen in her and hope she stabilizes. Then we'll move her. She opened her mouth to discuss things with Dr. Bernstein, but he was already sitting next to Victoria with her hand in his. Dr. Olson followed his lead and went back into the room. She joined them in mid-conversation.

"It just came on suddenly, doctor," Victoria was saying. "I feel like I'm suffocating now!"

"Okay, we can help you with that. Dr. Olson has called your daughter, and she's on her way. We're going to get you to intensive care, okay?"

"I just feel like I'm suffocating," Victoria repeated.

Dr. Olson watched the oxygen monitor. It was rising! Slowly, but it was going up! Thankful that they didn't need to intubate her this instant, she also knew it was imminent, and they were far from out of the woods. Dr. Bernstein's eyes were also on the monitor. He gave his colleague a quick nod and stood up.

"Get a blood gas and I'll call her in," he said on his way out of the room. This was code for "let's hope they have a bed available in the intensive care unit." Dr. Olson was amazed at how relaxed he seemed to be, and she couldn't help but feel envious.

Karen was flitting around the room, packing up Victoria's belongings in large plastic bags. Dr. Olson felt annoyed. The nurse's priority seemed was to get rid of this patient just as soon as possible. Dr. Olson's priority was to stabilize her. Relations between nurses and doctors could be a challenge, especially when the team had different priorities. They needed just a few minutes to monitor Victoria and get the blood work so they knew exactly what they were dealing with. It was difficult enough to get an arterial blood gas without having the added pressure of the nurse trying to wheel the patient out the door at lightning speed.

"Do you feel any better?" Dr. Olson asked Victoria. Her oxygen level was now 93 percent.

Victoria nodded.

"Good, I'm going to have to get an arterial blood gas now. Do you know what that is?"

Victoria shook her head.

"It's just like a regular blood test, except I won't use a tourniquet, and I get the blood out of this artery here, rather than the vein." She pointed to her own wrist.

Dr. Olson was good at this, but even so, arterial blood gases hurt. The artery is covered in nerves that the needle has to push through to get the blood, whereas the vein doesn't, so it hurts less. Dr. Olson left this part out of her explanation. The arterial blood gave more information about oxygen levels than the venous blood did, so there wasn't really much of a choice. She had to do it. She had to know how bad it really was.

Dr. Olson asked Karen if there was a blood gas kit in the room, and the nurse handed it to her without a word. The hostility was tangible, and Dr. Olson had to push it from her mind. She had to get the blood. She opened the kit and swabbed down Victoria's wrist with alcohol. She felt for the pulse, counted to three and stuck. Victoria didn't flinch. The blood flashed into the syringe, and within two seconds, it was all over. Dr. Olson breathed a sigh of relief that she had the precious blood gas.

"Can we move her now?" Karen asked.

"Dr. Bernstein is calling for a bed." Dr. Olson taped up Victoria's wrist and left the room.

At the nursing station, Dr. Bernstein had the phone to his ear and scribbled something on a piece of paper for Dr. Olson to read.

Bed 1271.

Just as Dr. Olson turned to tell the nurse that they had a bed in the unit, she saw Victoria's bed come wheeling into the hallway. Karen was on her cell and apparently, the nursing supervisor had already told her the news. With a shrug, Dr. Olson followed her patient down the hall.

As the nurses wheeled Victoria into her new room, Dr. Olson, Dr. Bernstein, and Lana, stood in the central nursing station in the intensive care unit. The beeps and chirps of ventilators and machines filled the room. The noise was shrill, and the nursing station looked like a command station with its monitors and computers. The glass walls revealed patients in other rooms, affording little to no privacy. Bright red metallic emergency carts sat poised outside the rooms, their very presence ominous.

The sterility of the unit struck Lana, but it was the strange noises that had caught her off guard as she'd entered the ICU. Now, she felt disoriented as she looked through the glass window to see her mom lying in a bed, wearing a mask that covered her face. She hadn't even had a moment to say hello to her mother before the doctors had pulled her aside. Lana felt overwhelmed.

The doctors knew it was time for the talk, the "code status" talk. Dr. Olson had briefed Lana about the cancer, but she still wasn't sure how much Lana *understood* about her mother's condition, so they started simply: they asked her.

"All I know is that three weeks ago, the only problem she had was that she was more tired than usual, and now, I hear that she's been diagnosed with colon cancer that has spread to her lung," Lana said.

"I think we should start by looking at her x-ray." Dr. Bernstein motioned Lana and Dr. Olson over to the computer.

Lana had no idea how to read an x-ray, and she was afraid she wouldn't understand what the doctors were showing her. She didn't say anything, though, and politely followed behind the doctors.

As soon as the computer loaded the film, Lana's hands rocketed up to cover her mouth, and she let out a loud gasp then yelled, "Oh my god!" Lana didn't know what she was looking at, but she knew that it was a big, white, round ball smack dab in the middle of her mom's x-ray. Smaller, irregular ones were all over the lungs.

Lana didn't know how to "read" an x-ray, but it didn't matter. You didn't have to go to medical school to understand this one. Quieter this time, Lana said, "I had no idea it was this bad. No idea."

Dr. Bernstein waited to let Lana compose herself. When she was ready, he explained what she was looking at. "As you can see, there is more tumor here than there is lung. But this one—this big ball here?—*this* is the problem."

Lana's eyes fell upon Dr. Olson, whose head was tilted to the side with sympathy. The sadness in Lana's eyes made the doctor feel two inches tall. She knew Lana could understand the picture in front of her, and she searched for words to comfort her, but none came.

Dr. Bernstein explained all that had happened in the last hour and pointed to the mass one more time, tracing it with his finger.

"This is *terminal* cancer, isn't it?" Lana looked over at Dr. Olson, who nodded. "This is going to kill her."

Dr. Olson was amazed at how quickly Lana understood and how effective showing her the x-ray had been. They had forgone the long conversation about obstructions and airways and lung tissue. It was all in the picture, and words could not have explained the situation better. Lana *got* it. She understood. They hadn't said much, but Dr. Olson felt that the three of them were all on the same level, the same page, and now, it was time to make the decisions.

"Let's go talk with her." Dr. Bernstein led the way back into Victoria's new room.

She's getting worse, thought Dr. Olson. Victoria's calm had dissolved into a panic. Her eyes were wide open, and she was gasping through the non-breather mask. The blood gas had revealed that her oxygen level was very low, and now that the mask was failing, it was time to put her on a breathing machine. Lana was already at her mother's side. She knew that Dr. Olson was the junior one of the two doctors, but for some reason, she kept looking to her for answers.

"We have a few options at this point." Dr. Olson directed her words at both Lana and Victoria, telling them the truth but as delicately as possible. "Obviously, she is very short of breath, and the mask isn't working well enough. The next step from here is to put a tube down into your lungs and hook you up to the breathing machine."

"Okay! Get the tube!" gasped Victoria. There was a new desperation in her voice.

"I can get the tube, but you have to understand that if we put the tube in, it might not be able to come out. I need you to understand that, and that you won't be able to speak." She paused before continuing. "The other option is that we can give you morphine to help slow your breathing and not put you on life support, but keep you as comfortable as possible."

"Get the tube!" gasped Victoria. Her eyes were wild and her voice unsteady.

Dr. Bernstein was concerned. The problem was that he knew from the chart that no one had discussed what Victoria's wishes were prior to this moment. And this was the *wrong* moment. Victoria couldn't make sound decisions in her state of air hunger. The next few moments were critical: they had to figure out what they would do *after* they put her on the machine. How long would Victoria want to be kept alive on a machine? Would she want them to perform CPR if her heart stopped? Would she want to be kept alive artificially? Would she want them to surgically place a feeding tube, since she wouldn't be able to eat once on the breathing machine? Or, would she want to be made comfortable, forgoing the intubation and the respirator? Would she prefer to be placed on medicine to calm her air hunger, but would certainly mean she would die in the next few hours? These were questions that Fred couldn't ask this woman in this state. It was already far too late.

"Get the tube!" gasped Victoria again.

Lana's eyes were steady though she was fighting back tears. She had to be strong for her mother. She had to keep her composure. This was neither the time nor the place to cry. She had to make sure that whatever was about to happen that she remained in control.

"Do you understand that you won't be able to tell us what your wishes are once we put you on the ventilator?" Dr. Olson asked, not realizing that she was actually shouting. The panic in Victoria's eyes made it obvious that the real Victoria, the calm Victoria was slipping away. Dr. Bernstein and Dr. Olson's eyes met. They were both concerned since this was not the ideal situation to be discussing end of life wishes.

Victoria's hand reached up to Lana. "You tell them what I want. You do it," panted Victoria as her hand dropped back down onto the bed from the exhaustion of the sentence.

Lana knew that her mom was finished talking. She knew what her mother was asking her to do. The question was to "suffocate," or not to "suffocate." That was it. It was not about ventilator machine or no machine. It was more primitive than that. Her mother did not want to die this way; she did not want to suffocate. She wanted air. She wanted to breathe.

Victoria was becoming restless and desperate and Lana realized that she had missed the window of opportunity to discuss with her mom about whether she would want to be sustained on life support. But right now, in this instant, Lana's first priority was to calm her mom, to make her more comfortable and to help her to relax.

She looked at her mother and swallowed: "Alright, Mom. We're getting the tube."

Dr. Olson stood in awe as she watched Victoria give her life over to Lana. It was terrifying and beautiful. Fred also saw the transfer, which in his medical mind, was that Victoria had just made Lana her "surrogate." Lana was now the decision maker.

"Please, help her breathe," Lana said to the doctors. "She is so uncomfortable. She needs to be peaceful and rest. Let's put her on the machine so she can be calm, and then we can decide later what we want to do."

With a nod, Fred spun around, poked his head out of the room and asked the nearest nurse to prepare for an emergent intubation.

Once Victoria was on the ventilator, Lana heaved a huge sigh of relief. The emergency was over. Her mother was breathing. Well, sort of. But at least she wasn't gasping. She was under sedation with a tube in her mouth that was connected to an enormous mysterious box, the ventilator. Lana had time now. She had time to figure this out.

She headed for the family waiting area and collapsed with a sigh into one of the chairs. She reached into her purse and pulled out her cell phone, not sure which one of her seven siblings to call first. She knew Sara would have the hardest time with the news that Mom was on life support, being the youngest and also the closest to Mom. She dialled her oldest brother first and the phone chain began from there. Within a few hours, the entire family was on their way to the hospital. They were a large group, and Lana didn't know how everyone would react. Lana always thought of her family as more of a cast of characters than as a close-knit group. They all had their own personalities, their own lives, their own interests, so gathering everyone together under such a devastating condition was a situation that filled Lana with angst. How would she get everyone to come together? What would she say? What if they started arguing? How could she control the situation? Would they be able to unite as a family and make a single, coherent decision? Lana was doubtful and put her head in her hands as she waited for their arrival.

Sara was the first to arrive and Lana was thankful that she intercepted her before she was able to see Victoria on the ventilator. Lana knew she had to prepare Sara for what she was going to see. She had to slow her down, to get her rational, and Sara arrived dishevelled, obviously having rushed out the door when she had heard of the intubation. After a few quick hugs and an update, Lana took Sara inside the ICU to see Victoria, wondering just how many times she'd have to intercept family members to prepare them for what they would see.

Victoria was the figurehead of their family, the single unifying theme. She was pragmatic and strong, never vulnerable. But now, sedated on the medications and intubated, she had the fragility of a porcelain doll. It was hard to prepare for and even harder to see. Lana had to relive the agony of seeing her mother so vulnerable with every new arrival.

Finally, after the entire family had gathered, Victoria's doctors approached Lana about holding a family meeting, one in which they could explain the recent events to the family members who had gathered in the waiting room. Lana was relieved that someone else was going to do the explaining and together, Lana and her mother's doctors herded the group into the family conference room.

The room, although spacious, seemed to collapse under the weight of the forty-some family members who had gathered there. Despite the large group, the silence was deafening in the room as the last of the family filed in. Lana, Sara, Dr. Olson, and Dr. Bernstein were the only ones to sit, while the rest of the family crowded around Lana and Sara in a group. It was the oldest and the youngest, flanked by all those in between. Dr. Olson looked around the room and saw one tear-streaked face after the next until her eyes fell upon Lana, who remained calm and pragmatic, the new figurehead and the obvious leader of the group.

Dr. Bernstein began. "Thank you all for coming here. I know this is really hard. It's wonderful to see everyone coming together, though, and I'm not sure we've ever had a group this large in here before." Soft chuckles rolled through the room.

"As I guess you all know by now," he continued, "Victoria has terminal cancer, and earlier today, we had to place her on the ventilator to help her breathe, and its unlikely at this time that she will be able to come off because of the amount of tumor that is obstructing her air tube."

He paused. Dr. Olson surveyed the room once more and saw nothing but stillness.

"We need to make some decisions about where to go from here, but since there are so many of you, I first want to make sure that we are all on the same page about who is going to be the main decision maker." Dr. Bernstein looked cautiously at Lana, hoping that the group knew that Lana had already assumed the responsibility.

"Yes," Lana said, "we've already established that I am going to be the voice of the group, that I will be the decision maker, but I'm going to be discussing everything with all the siblings." Heads nodded in agreement.

"Good. That is exactly what we'd like to happen. We want everyone to speak his or her mind and be involved, but we do need to assign someone as the decision maker, and it was pretty clear that your mom wanted you, Lana, to do that.

"From here, we have to make decisions about how aggressive we are going to be regarding her care. First, she has an incurable cancer. It seems you all understand that. Am I correct in saying that?"

Heads nodded, and some quiet sobs could be heard from the back.

"Did Victoria ever talk to any of you about her end-of-life wishes or her feelings about life support, things like that?" Fred asked, hopeful that someone from the crowd would speak up.

There was silence until Lana spoke. "No. I mean, she wasn't sick. We never talked about it, or really even though about it."

"Was anyone close to Victoria ever really sick or on life support?" Dr. Olson asked, "Did she ever experience having a friend or family member critically ill?"

"Her cousin had a stroke years ago, but I don't think Victoria was all that involved in the details," an older woman offered.

"All right, so, we don't really know how she would feel about being on life support," Dr. Bernstein concluded. "We'll have to move forward making assumptions, unfortunately, based on the things you know to be true of Victoria's feelings and things that are important to her.

"This cancer is pretty extensive. The amount of tumor in her lungs concerns me that it will be difficult, if not impossible, for us to get her off the ventilator, and even if we do get her off, it will be challenging to keep her off. So, knowing this, I think it's best to start talking about what our goals are, what we'd like to achieve, and what we *can* reasonably achieve." He paused. There was stillness in the room and no one seemed to want to say anything, so he continued.

"Different people have different goals, and so if we can talk for a moment about your mom's lifestyle, the things she found important in her life, what quality of life meant for her," Fred said with an encouraging expression for others to speak up.

"She is incredibly independent," Lana said. "She's always insisted on doing everything herself and has always resisted offers to assist her with just about anything, even just getting out of a car." Chuckles fanned out in the room.

"She is a stubborn one," an elderly woman added with a tone of affection.

Dr. Bernstein and Dr. Olson smiled, and the room softened as Victoria's family members exchanged stories about Victoria's unrelenting independence.

Dr. Olson listened and admired the family before her, seeing how their faces lightened as they told stories about Victoria and the things she enjoyed doing.

"She loved the boardwalk," Sara offered. "It always made me nervous when she'd go out there alone, but she wouldn't hear of it otherwise. Walking the boardwalk was one of her favorite things to do. In fact . . ." Her voice trailed away as she began digging through her purse and pulled out a wallet of photographs and flipped to one and handed it across to Dr. Bernstein.

Dr. Olson looked over his shoulder at the image of a younger Victoria sitting on a bench at what appeared to be the Atlantic City Boardwalk. She was wearing a grey spring coat and matching hat with a serious but happy expression on her face.

"I took that photo with a disposable camera Mom had just bought for me, back when disposable cameras were brand new," Sara said.

Dr. Olson smiled broadly at the photograph and looked up to see how Victoria's family's posture and dynamics had changed. Arms were uncrossed, and the faces seemed softer and less afraid.

"Thanks for sharing that, Sara." Dr. Bernstein passed the photo back to Sara, who handed it off into the crowd behind her, and they began passing it around.

"From what I'm hearing," Dr. Bernstein began, "Victoria was an independent woman, so I have to question whether the idea of long-term life support is something she would want."

"She would definitely not want to live the rest of her life on life support," Lana said resolutely. Others nodded their heads in agreement.

"So, this leaves us in a difficult spot. We have to make some decisions about how to move forward and how we're going to best uphold what we think Victoria would want us to do for her," Dr. Bernstein said.

"How long, do you think she has left, doctor?" a voice from the crowd asked.

"Well, that really depends on how we move forward," Fred said, "on life support, we might be able to keep her alive for quite some time. I mean, she doesn't have any infections or any immediate catastrophes threatening her life, other than her cancer, of course. The ventilator is working well, so the effects of the cancer are tempered right now by the tube in her throat and the machine helping her get oxygen in and get carbon dioxide out, which is what we call ventilation. She is ventilating well, but only because we have her on the machine. If we were to remove it, I'm not entirely sure how long she would live, but I would suspect it would not be for very long."

"This just happened so fast," Lana said. "I just wish we could talk to her."

"I know it's hard. Right now, we have her on a good dose of sedatives to keep her pain-free, but as a result of that, she is unaware of what's going on around her. If we lighten those up, she'd wake up a little, but she'd also be pretty uncomfortable from the tube in her throat."

Dr. Olson saw that Lana and most of her family were vehemently shaking their heads no.

"Before we make any decisions about the ventilator and about life support, let's talk first about our goals here, knowing we can't cure her, or make her the independent woman she used to be," Dr. Bernstein said.

Sara spoke up. "I'd like to be able to talk to her, but I guess that would mean taking her off the machine, which I don't think we should do yet."

Dr. Olson looked at Lana, who looked down at her hands on the table.

"Is it possible for her to get off the machine, so she can talk to us?" Lana asked.

"We can certainly try to do that," Fred said, adding "and I think that is a reasonable goal in this situation. If we try to wean her off the ventilator and get the tube out, we'll be able to control her pain without the heavy doses of narcotics she needs on the vent, yet still control any symptoms that may come up, like shortness of breath or pain, by using morphine."

"How long will that take?" Sara asked.

Dr. Bernstein looked to Dr. Olson. "What was her last blood gas like?"

"It was good. We have her oxygen and carbon dioxide levels controlled, but we still haven't figured out why she had the acute episode," Dr. Olson said cautiously. She knew that in order to figure out why Victoria had all of a sudden had acute shortness of breath, they would need to order a battery of tests in hopes of finding some reversible cause for the sudden decline. Something other than the plain fact that she had cancer filling her lungs.

"Right. So, what Dr. Olson is saying is that although we know her chronic problem is her cancer, the acute problem that caused her to get put on the ventilator may be from something else, like perhaps a blood clot in her lung."

"And is that something that you could fix?" Sara asked, hope filling her voice.

"No, but we'd have to first get a CT scan of her lungs to see if she even has one, and if so, we could start a blood thinner to prevent it from getting worse, but blood clots really only go away with time. And with the blood thinner, we run into risks of bleeding and whatnot," he explained.

Dr. Olson clenched her teeth. Beginning a work-up for a blood clot, or a pulmonary embolism, would complicate matters and likely wouldn't change the outcome for the better.

"So, if you started this medication, it wouldn't impact whether she got off the ventilator?" Lana asked.

"Correct," Fred replied. "We could look for other causes of this shortness of breath, hoping to find something reversible, perhaps something cardiac—"

Lana raised her hand to interrupt. "I don't see the point in putting her through a CT scan and all that. It's not going to change matters. I saw her x-ray," Lana said firmly, looking over at Sara, who nodded feebly in agreement.

"I think that's a reasonable decision," Dr. Olson offered. "If our goal is get her off the ventilator, we should focus on that."

"Right," Dr. Bernstein agreed. "Are we all in agreement?"

The heads in the room nodded. Lana confirmed, "Let's just try and get her off the ventilator so she can talk to us and see us."

"Okay, good," he answered. "We have a clear goal then. That's what we're going to work toward. In the meantime, there a few other things we need to consider: for example, what might happen if she were to suddenly decline or if her heart were to stop beating? We could attempt to resuscitate her with CPR or electric shocks to restart her heart, but even if we were successful, we'd be in the same position we are now, but we'd have the added damage from the CPR itself and the results of however long the heart didn't pump blood to her brain and vital organs." After a short pause to take his measure of the room, he added "I think that would make things a lot worse."

Dr. Olson held her breath. This was the DNR decision, whether or not to give the doctors the instruction, "do not resuscitate." She felt strongly that resuscitating Victoria, or coding her, would be overly aggressive, and she imagined herself having to do chest compressions or shocks and threading long IV catheters into Victoria's groin as was common during a code. She hoped with all hope that they said no.

"Well, if it happened before you got her off the ventilator and you restarted her heart, we might still be able to talk to her, so I think you should at least try," Sara said quickly.

Dr. Olson's heart sank. Sara, she suspected, was imaging CPR like she's seen on television, the kind where the patient receives CPR and before the show is over is the patient is up chasing bad guys or whatever the case may be. It's an overly optimistic view. Never during these shows do they depict the central line being stuck into the groin to administer the code medications. It never shows the ventilator being placed, which must always occur with CPR. They don't show the red scorch marks where the shocks are delivered to the chest, nor do they play the sound of the ribs cracking. Never do they address the high likelihood of brain damage if CPR continues for a long period of time, and how we sometimes begin a post-cardiac arrest period of hypothermia to reduce the likelihood of brain damage. Typically, hypothermia comes with a twenty-four hour period when the body is chilled down to temperatures so cold that paralytic medications are used to prevent the violent shivering that results. Television and media often neglect to address these realities.

"For some patients, Sara," Fred began, "CPR can be quite successful. But in patients with end-stage, terminal conditions, the chances of it helping, rather than hurting, is incredibly low. My honest opinion is that CPR would do nothing except prolong the period in which your mother is dying, and wouldn't put us any closer to our goal of getting her off the ventilator."

"No CPR, no shocks," Lana said. "If it's going to restart her heart just to keep her alive like this, then I don't see the point."

Dr. Olson looked around to try and get a feel of what the crowd thought of Lana's decision. Sara had buried her face in her hands for a moment, but then nodded in agreement..

Fred continued. "I think that's a really reasonable and appropriate decision, Lana. From here we can do one of two things in regards to getting her off the ventilator. We can take her off today, with morphine to control any pain or shortness of breath, or we can give it a few days and see if we can wean her gradually and see how she does."

It was at this point in the meeting that Dr. Olson saw the stoic faces begin to really react to the information. Twisted faces and tears filled the room whilst arms came from seemingly nowhere to embrace each other.

Sara leaned onto Lana, who kept her eyes on Dr. Olson, whose facial expression kept her at ease. Lana could feel Dr. Olson comforting her silently, and Lana knew Dr. Olson would be there to help her face the looming decisions.

"It's possible that we could get her off the ventilator with just a few days of weaning trials," Dr. Bernstein said. "She'd have to have a nice slow breathing rate and we'd have to lift the sedation to make her alert enough to breath on her own before taking the tube out, but it's also possible that we won't be able to remove the sedation easily if the pain causes her to breathe fast or panic. It can be challenging, and sometimes a lengthy process, especially in situations like these. It's really up to you to think about what duration of life support, if any, you think your mom would agree to."

"And if we took her off today, she'd probably die today?" asked a woman in the back.

"Probably," Dr. Olson said gently, "although, it's hard to know for sure. She isn't ready to breathe on her own yet, but if we took the tube out, we'd use the medications to keep her comfortable and pain-free. Perhaps she'd wake up after the tube came out and we fine-tuned her medications, but there's a chance she wouldn't. It's hard to say. Either direction you choose, we would do everything we could to limit her discomfort."

"I hear what you're saying. I just . . . well . . ." Lana gathered her thoughts. "I guess we will need a little time as a family to discuss it and decide . . . I mean, we want her off the machine. I just don't know if we're ready to do it today." Lana's eyes searched Dr. Olson's face as if looking for some sort of hint as to what she should do.

"By all means, take some time to yourselves," Dr. Bernstein answered. "And if you want to talk more, Dr. Olson and I will be in the unit."

Lana nodded as the doctors stood to leave. Dr. Olson lingered for a moment because she felt awkward leaving Lana behind. "I'll be right outside if you have any questions." She looked straight at Lana.

Dr. Olson slipped out of the room and the door clicked quietly behind her. Sobs erupted as she walked away from the meeting room, and she headed back to the unit to sit and wait for their decision.

Forty-five minutes passed before Lana made her way back into the ICU to look for Dr. Olson, who was sitting behind the desk at the nurse's station. The doctor rose when she saw Lana enter the unit and met her as she approached.

"How are you?" Dr. Olson asked, the concern in her voice real and sincere.

"I'm actually okay," Lana said. "We just have to take what comes, I guess."

"I'm so sorry you are in this situation."

"Thank you. It's very hard, but I feel like Mom is getting good care, and I cannot thank you enough for that. I can really tell that you care about us, and it means a lot to me."

Dr. Olson reached out and touched Lana's arm. "You are most welcome. Your mother reminds me of my own mother, and so it's especially hard for me to watch everything that is happening. I really feel for you and want to help in any way I can."

The two women stood in a silent bond for a few seconds before Dr. Olson asked, "Have you decided?"

"We want to give it a few days and see how she does on the ventilator. Sara is hoping that she might wake up a little and be able to communicate with us once she settles down on the ventilator. She is really not ready to take her off the ventilator, although some of my other siblings are leaning in that direction. But, we decided that for now, we'd like to keep the machine going," Lana said.

"That's a fine plan," Dr. Olson replied. "We'll keep the ventilator going but will not attempt CPR or shocks, like we talked about earlier. It would also be helpful for me to know how to react if her blood pressure drops or if her oxygen levels were to drop." Dr. Olson's mind raced through all the foreseeable possibilities. She wanted to be absolutely sure that she knew what Lana and her family wanted should something happen in the middle of the night. "If her blood pressure were to drop, we could start medications to keep it up, but truthfully, those kinds of medications would just be prolonging the dying process in this situation."

"No, if she starts to slip away, just let her go." Lana's words rang resolute and confident. "I know she isn't going to get better, but I guess we are all hoping that perhaps in a few days she might get to the point where she can hear us, or even communicate with us if that's possible."

"Of course. We'll do whatever we can to try and make that happen." Dr. Olson wasn't particularly hopeful that they would be successful, but she would do her best. "We'll take it one day at a time. Remember, you can always change your mind later, and we can revisit this if need be."

"All right, thanks," Lana said. With a sad but satisfied smile, she left to sit by her mother's side.

Five days later, Dr. Olson popped her head into Victoria's room to give her a quick look. The intern had written the daily note, and Dr. Olson had not yet had a chance to do her daily check on Victoria's condition. She was happy to find Lana at the bedside, but was taken aback at how upset she looked.

"Hi," she said, trying to mix cheer and empathy into her voice. "How are you doing?"

Lana wiped her emotions from her face and answered, "I'm okay. She just looks awful!" Over the last five days, Victoria hadn't even opened her eyes, let alone communicated with anyone. She hadn't given any sign that she had any awareness of their presence, and that had been devastating to the whole family. The weaning attempts had not been successful, and there wasn't much sign of improvement.

Lana paused to look at her mother before continuing. "She seems to be wasting away, and her eyes are sunken. She's looking worse and worse every day."

Dr. Olson knew that this might be Lana's turning point and could tell by the look on her face that the decision to take Victoria off the ventilator could be at hand.

"You're right." Dr. Olson's voice stayed even and soft. "She is becoming quite frail, but hemodynamically, she is still stable."

"She's not weaning at all, is she?" Lana asked, already knowing the answer.

"No." The word carried her apology.

"I just think she has fought so hard, and she looks so tired," Lana said. "It's tough to see her looking like this."

Dr. Olson said nothing but leaned forward to encourage Lana to continue talking.

"It's been really hard for my sister Sara; she is really close to Mom. And Sara will never be able to say 'stop,' although I know that is what she is thinking."

"What do *you* think?" Dr. Olson studied Lana's face. "Regardless of what the rest of your family says, you first have to make up your own mind about what you think you should do."

Without hesitation, Lana said, "I think she is too tired and it's time for her to rest. She has put in a hard fight, but look at her! She wouldn't want this: she wouldn't want to live the rest of her life on the ventilator."

"So you feel like we should discontinue the ventilator?" Dr. Olson asked, conscious of the fact that she was uttering the words that most families have such a hard time saying.

"Yes, I do." Lana spoke evenly.

"And you are worried that Sara is going to have a hard time agreeing to it?"

"Exactly." Lana sighed.

The two women stood silently, surrounded by the humming of the ventilator as it pushed breath into Victoria's diseased lungs.

Lana made up her mind. "I'm going to talk to the family after lunch today and try to get an idea of where everyone is. But I'm pretty sure that the family is coming to terms with the fact that Mom is fighting a losing battle."

"Well, this is just a different way to look at it, but perhaps if she passes with the whole family with her, perhaps that is a way in which she can win," Dr. Olson suggested.

Lana shook her head in agreement and let out another soft sigh.

"I'll be right outside if you need me." Dr. Olson slid quietly out of the room.

A few hours later, Lana had gathered the family in the waiting area and was waiting for Dr. Bernstein to come outside and give them the okay to come into the unit. There were nearly forty of them again, so the unit had to make some special preparations to accommodate everyone at once. They moved all the unnecessary equipment and waste bins outside of the room and cleared an area outside of Victoria's room for the overflow of people. They had pushed the ventilator and IV poles as close to the wall as they could, to allow for the most people to fit in the room.

Dr. Bernstein emerged from the double doors, and they whooshed shut behind him. "We're ready for you now," he said to Lana.

"Okay. Thank you, doctor, for letting all of us come in to be with her," Lana said appreciatively. She was well aware that normally only two visitors at a time were allowed. "It means a lot to us."

"Of course. It's not a problem at all. We want to accommodate everyone who wants to be here. You can head in whenever you are ready."

Lana motioned to her siblings to follow Fred into the unit, but she stayed behind so that she could walk in with Sara, whom she knew was hanging toward the back of the crowd.

Lana talked with her sister once it was just the two of them. "You okay, Sara?"

"No."

"I know this is tough, but she isn't going to get better. You know that, right?"

"Yeah." Sara stared at the floor.

"Are you going to be able to go through with this?"

"No. I can't say the words, Lana. I can't say that I want to take her off life support. I won't say it!" Sara burst into tears.

"You don't have to, Sis. I will say it. I just need to know that you won't hate me for it," Lana said, hugging her little sister.

"No, I don't hate you!" Sara laughed through her tears.

"Come on, then. Let's go," Lana said, pulling Sara towards the door. "You don't have to say anything at all."

Dr. Olson had never seen so many people crammed into a patient's room. It felt like a cartoon, in a way, with people piled on top of one another and spilling out into the main unit. Dr. Bernstein was in the room, as there needed to be only one physician for the withdrawal of the ventilator, so Dr. Olson stayed outside, watching through the glass window.

Lana and Sara were at the head of the bed with the doctor and the respiratory therapist. Victoria's nurse had hung a morphine drip several minutes earlier, and the medication was permeating in Victoria's veins by now. She hadn't seemed to be breathless or in pain without the morphine drip, but it was standard to have it going, just in case the breathlessness emerged. The room was quiet except for the sobs and the sounds of the monitors and machines.

Dr. Bernstein nodded to the respiratory technician who unstrapped the collar that held the ventilator tube in place. As he loosened the chinstrap, they could see the indentations in Victoria's chin. With one slow and steady motion, he pulled the tube lightly until it was entirely out of Victoria's mouth. Loud alarms erupted from the ventilator box as it detected that the tube had come out. The technician reached over quickly to silence it. He then took a suction catheter and cleared the saliva that had pooled in her mouth. Once the tube was out, Victoria's jaw closed gently for the first time since she had been intubated. She was breathing in tiny, shallow breaths. Her eyes remained closed, and her body was still. Fred was relieved that there was no sudden gasp for air, which happens occasionally during an extubation, something that usually upsets the family. Instead, Victoria was peaceful and serene, the way the family remembered her, her mouth closed, no tubes jutting out. She was as close to the mother that Lana had known as was possible. Instead of the sounds of the ventilator, the soft whispers of prayers emanated from the crowd in the room, and the family stood together with Victoria as her breathing slowed.

Outside, Dr. Olson wondered how long it would take. She had performed many terminal extubations and was amazed at how different each one could be. Some patients linger for hours after the ventilator is withdrawn. They're able to breath on their own for a few hours, but eventually, the strength that allowed them to maintain their oxygen levels fades and they succumb to a respiratory fatigue. Others go right away, as they simply cannot survive for any length of time without the ventilator. Dr. Olson wondered what Victoria's body would do and then wondered which way would be *best*. Is it easier for the family if the patient dies right away so they don't have to stand by and watch a long and drawn out decline? Yet, when it happens right after the ventilator is withdrawn, it might worsen feelings of guilt because the family sees a direct relation to *their* decision to take out the tube and the death of their loved one. Dr. Olson sometimes thought it was better if the two events were spaced out in time, but you could never be sure how any family will react to the passing of loved one. It always seemed to be a little easier when the family had some time with their loved one after they were unveiled from the shroud of the ventilator. Dr. Olson hoped Victoria could breathe on her own long enough for all forty of her family members to say their goodbyes in their own time.

Victoria passed away within twenty minutes. As her shallow breaths could not sustain her oxygen levels, her heart eventually slowed and ceased to beat. Her death was gentle and peaceful, and her final moments were spent surrounded by the ones who loved her most. She felt no pain and her family stood on as a unit as they said their goodbyes. There was no CPR, no drama, simply peace. Victoria's death was neat and organized, just like the home that she kept. There was no chaos or uncertainty, but instead there were prayers and love.

Lana and Sara were the last in the room after the nurse switched off the monitor. At the time her heart had stopped, they had all seen it on the monitor, and Dr. Bernstein had gone inside the room to declare Victoria deceased. As the family trickled out one by one, Dr. Olson waited in the nursing station, hoping for a moment to say goodbye to Lana. She reflected on her first meeting with Victoria and remembered her calm eyes, how they had reminded her of her own mother's. She recalled how important it had been for her to "get it right" with Victoria's care. Looking back on the whole experience, Dr. Olson knew that they had. Victoria's death had matched her personality: calm and contained. They had enabled her entire family to be at her bedside and controlled the situation enough so that everyone could be at peace.

Sara left the room, her face streaked with tears, and Lana came out a few seconds behind her. She saw Dr. Bernstein was in the room across the way, speaking with the family member of another patient. Her eyes searched for Dr. Olson and she found her sitting in the nursing station. She approached her with a smile.

"Thank you for everything," Lana said.

"You are most welcome," Dr. Olson said. "Your mother was a very brave woman."

Lana sniffed and nodded but did not cry. Her eyes were calm and steady, a glimpse into Victoria's strength, passed on to her daughter.

"Take care," Dr. Olson said.

"I will," Lana said. As she turned to leave, she took one last look at Dr. Olson and at the unit. With a nod to herself, she pushed through the door without looking back.

* * *

I wasn't involved in Victoria's care, but one of my best friends, "Dr. Olson," was. As she told me of her experience meeting and caring for Victoria, what struck me most about the story was the way she spoke of Victoria's daughter, Lana. She talked about Lana's eyes, her demeanor, and the way she just seemed to "get it." Dr. Olson confided in me that she felt a deep connection to Lana, as if they had known each other for years.

Two weeks after Dr. Olson shared this story with me, I interviewed Lana. She spoke of "that female doctor," the one who was there, the one with the kind eyes and the warm personality. She talked about the details of her mother's hospital stay with impressive medical knowledge and an enviable composure, but her tone changed from facts to feelings whenever she mentioned Dr. Olson. She remembered even the smallest of gestures, a head tilt or simple body language. The bond between these two women was completely reciprocated. They both spoke of the other's eyes using almost identical words. I was envious of the connection.

I often feel attached to my patients' families, but equally often wonder if I am deluding myself. Am I really making a difference in a time when there seems to be no way to really make an impact or alleviate a stranger's grief? Lana and Dr. Olson spoke about each other during their interviews almost as much as they talked about Victoria, making me realize that the relationship between the doctors and families are just as important, if not more so, than I had come to believe.

"Dr. Olson slowed down when she felt I needed her to slow down," Lana said. "She went at my pace, not her own pace, so that I would truly understand what was going on." Although Lana knew and remembered the precise medical details of how her mother's disease progressed, it was the people surrounding her, the doctors and her family, that really positively impacted the way she experienced her mother's death.

Lana has no regrets with the way the events unfolded. To her, it was perfect. Yet I felt sympathy that Lana had had to assume the medical decisions for her mother so suddenly and without any preparation. She'd found herself suddenly a surrogate decision maker, a proxy; in the end, she'd had to decide what her mother would most want regarding her medical care and end-of-life experience.

Dr. Olson told me how Lana handled the stress and burden with ease and grace, despite the fact that she hadn't had end-of-life conversations or preparations with her mother prior to this emergency. This fascinated me. How could someone who had virtually no preparation and no prior warning handle end-of-life decisions for another person with such apparent ease? When I asked Lana the question she had a simple answer.

"Put yourself on the side," she told me. "It's not about what you want; it's about what your loved one wants." And the rest came easily.

Lana also emphasized to me the experience made her realize just how truly important it is to communicate with your family. "My mother's experience made me talk to my own children about my own end-of-life wishes." I smiled to myself as she spoke, her words resonating deeply because her lesson learned was exactly the one I hoped to spread by writing Victoria's story. "I want my kids to know how I would want to be cared for if something similar were to happen to me."

The unfortunate truth, however, is that you cannot predict your own story. None of us hold the crystal ball. Most of us choose not to think about things that are hard to confront, perhaps because of avoidance, denial, or fear. I challenge you to move past this hesitancy and consider your own story and wishes, and prepare yourself and your family as best as possible. Although Lana handled her dilemma with impressive composure, I've seen equally capable family members crumble under the stress. We owe it to those we love to do everything we can to circumvent any extra grief they experience during time of medical crisis.

My challenge to you may seem overwhelming, perhaps impossible, but the final chapter of *Last Wish* is a Resource Section, designed specifically for you to help navigate the feelings, emotions and questions you may have developed while reading the stories of these five incredible people.

Discussion Questions

1. Victoria's family was faced with an unexpected decision in a crisis situation. What would you have done if you were her daughters?

2. Ultimately, Victoria's family was guided by her values and preferences when it came to medical decision-making—what would you want your family to consider?

3. Modern medicine can keep the human body functioning in the setting of very serious illness, however just because we can intervene, does it mean we always should? What are the costs to patients, their families and the healthcare system?

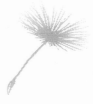

Resource Section:
Your Last Wish

Now you've vicariously experienced some of the more common medical decisions that you or your loved one may someday face. Most of the patients and families I've met through my work have not been exposed to any of these topics, and it is my hope that reading these stories has given you an advantage and insight into the world within the intensive care unit. Each story was chosen to demonstrate a specific concept, whether that is what CPR is truly like, what being on a breathing machine entails, what it's like to remove someone from life support, or the possible benefits of hospice care. Although at times, *LAST WISH* is admittedly tough to read, I hope that you have formed opinions and preferences about how you envision your own medical care to proceed should you become critically ill, whether that be full, aggressive care or one that is aimed more at comfort than cure.

Using these opinions, I encourage you to plan ahead and think about the topics and concepts presented in *LAST WISH*. An excellent way to begin this process is to complete an advance directive and name someone you know and trust as your surrogate decision maker (your power of attorney). What follows is a discussion about the times when these documents are helpful, and even more important, the times when they are not. Misconceptions of advance directives abound among doctors and patients alike, and it is my hope that this section can be used as a tool to provide some much-needed clarification.

Advance Directives:
Even Doctors Get It Wrong

My first lesson in advance directives snuck up on me when I was least expecting it. It was my second week in the intensive care unit, and my white coat was still pristine and freshly pressed. When I responded to a nurse yelling for assistance, I found myself in the precarious position of being the first doctor in the room for a cardiac arrest. As the nurse was scrambling for the oxygen mask, I started CPR. After a few minutes, the rest of the code team came crashing into the room, the patient was intubated and started on medications to raise the blood pressure. Once the patient's doctor arrived, he told us that the patient was seventy years old, never sick a day in his life, and had come in to the hospital with a pneumonia.

It wasn't very long before we had gotten back the pulse and the blood pressure. The patient was saved. As we stood around the patient's bedside, watching the monitor, a nurse came into the room waving a piece of paper. It was the patient's advance directive. On it was a checklist where the patient had checked off that he did not want CPR or mechanical ventilation. I remember how my heart dropped when I saw that paper. I had been the first to start CPR, and the thought never even occurred to me to even ask if the patient was a full code. I had just started the compressions.

I backed out of the room, my presence not missed amongst the swarms of more senior doctors who had since flooded the room since I had started the CPR. I welled up with tears, feeling horrified that I had done the wrong thing. I had started a code on a patient who was DNR. I ran down six flights of stairs to visit my mentor, Dr. Poe, and choked back tears as I plopped myself down onto my favorite chair in his office, one I would come to know often through the years.

Through my sobs, I told him what had happened and what I had done, but he just shook his head and grinned.

"Did you actually read the advance directive?" he asked me.

"Well, yeah," I moaned. "He checked off that he didn't want CPR or intubation."

"Did you read the statements before that?"

I didn't know what he was talking about, so I just kept right on crying, feeling terrible about what had happened. Once he calmed me down, he explained to me that I had in fact, done the right thing.

"This is exactly why I don't have an advance directive," he counselled. "No one understands them. This is a perfect example. You're a doctor and the advance directive confused you. From what you've told me, L. J., his advance directive doesn't apply. You did the right thing by saving him."

And he was right. I had done the right thing by starting the CPR, and he ended up walking out of the hospital just a few weeks later. Thankfully, the nurse brought in the advance directive *after* I had started the CPR. The confusion and more important, the lesson, is all about those first few statements, the ones no one ever reads or understands.

The Advance Directive Checklist:
yes/no....maybe

Unfortunately, even the most well-intentioned advance directive may be written in such a way that it can be incredibly difficult to interpret. Even the layout of the document can lead to a misinterpretation of what's written. And, obviously, when dealing with life and death, there's no room for misinterpretation. Below is an example of a common version of an advance directive; in fact, the same version that sent me weeping to Dr. Poe's office.

DECLARATION

I,_____, being of sound mind, willfully and voluntarily make this declaration to be followed if I become incompetent. This declaration reflects my firm and settled commitment to refuse life-sustaining treatment under the circumstances indicated below.

I direct my attending physician to withhold or withdraw life-sustaining treatment that serves only to prolong the process of my dying, if I should be in a terminal condition or in a state of permanent unconsciousness.

I direct that treatment be limited to measures to keep me comfortable and to relieve pain, including any pain that might occur by withholding or withdrawing life-sustaining treatment.

In addition, if I am in the condition described above, I feel especially strongly about the following forms of treatment:

I ( )do ( )do not want cardiac resuscitation.

I ( )do ( )do not want mechanical respiration.

I ( )do ( )do not want tube feeding or any other artificial or invasive form of nutrition (food) or hydration (water).

I ( )do ( )do not want blood or blood products.

I ( )do ( )do not want any form of surgery or invasive diagnostic tests.

I ( )do ( )do not want kidney dialysis.

I ( )do ( )do not want antibiotics.

I realize that if I do not specifically indicate my preference regarding any of the forms of treatment listed previously, I may receive that form of treatment.

The checklist draws our eyes immediately to the "Do/Do Not want" options. This can lead to inadvertently ignoring the most critical statement of all, the clause that lays out the condition in which the advance directive would take effect:

"I direct my attending physician to withhold or withdraw life-sustaining treatment that serves only to prolong the process of my dying *if I should be in a terminal condition or in a state of permanent unconsciousness.*"

Let's take for example two extremes to illustrate the importance of this statement. First, imagine that you were stung by a bee and had a terrible allergic reaction. You're otherwise healthy and perfectly fine, but allergic to bees. By the time you make it to the emergency room, your throat has swollen up and you can't breathe. The bee sting caused the swelling, which can be controlled and reversed by intravenous steroids and other medications, but these medications may take some time to work. The doctors need to put you on a ventilator or else you will die. You have a reversible condition requiring life support. Under this circumstance, the above advance directive doesn't apply.

This is crucial to understand: having an advance directive where you've checked off the box saying you would not want life support *does not mean* that you won't end up getting CPR or being put on a breathing machine if it is thought that your condition may be reversible or if it is unclear whether it is irreversible. There are certainly times when CPR or brief periods on life support can be life saving and beneficial, and advance directives are written in such a way to account for these situations, such as the bee sting. However, if your preference is to never, under any circumstances be put on life support, then this must be clearly specified in an advance directive and the wording of the generic advance directive would have to be changed.

Now let's look at the other extreme; for example, a patient like Victoria, whose terminal lung cancer caused her to develop shortness of breath so severe she required the ventilator in order to maintain her oxygen levels. She did not have an advance directive, and even though she had an irreversible condition, she was placed on life support. Had Victoria possessed an advance directive saying she would not want to be placed on a ventilator if she had an irreversible disease, she may have avoided being placed on the ventilator at the time of her respiratory de-compensation, had that been her wish. Instead, the doctors would have transitioned her care to palliative measures or hospice care, with an emphasis on administering medications to reduce her pain, discomfort and shortness of breath. When the decision about life support needed to be made emergently, Victoria was under too much duress to think clearly and make any decisions about her wishes, so she relied on Lana, her daughter, to make a decision without knowing what her mom may have wanted.

In situations like these, the advance directive may take some of the guesswork and decision making burden away from family members in emergent situations where clear thinking is seemingly impossible. It also may have helped Sara, Victoria's youngest daughter as she struggled with the final decision to remove Victoria from the ventilator. Perhaps an advance directive may have helped Sara come to terms with the ultimate decision to withdraw life support had she known it was truly her mother's own wish as documented in her advance directive.

Similarly, the drama, tension, and conflict that surrounded Mrs. Chandler's care might have been minimized had there been an advance directive. For Mrs. Chandler, the physicians felt that pressing on was inhumane, yet her family felt that Mrs. Chandler would have wanted every possible intervention to prolong her life, regardless of the state she was in. Missing from the whole dynamic was the voice of Mrs. Chandler. An advance directive could have confirmed her wishes, letting us know if she *did* in fact want fully aggressive care or something else. This could have alleviated much of the angst and tension between the medical team and the family and led to a better quality of care for Mrs. Chandler.

Advance Directives: Helpful to a Point

Advance directives can be incredibly useful when making decisions about what to do for a patient with a well-defined condition, like the bee sting or the end-stage lung cancer. However, try as we might to plan ahead for the end of life, the stark reality of it all is that decisions come up that we did not foresee. Our bodies are unpredictable, and so are the ways in which they will break down. Inevitably, there will be times when the advance directive can't predict a medical scenario that may present itself. There may be reversible processes superimposed on an irreversible one, for example, a pneumonia in a patient with breast cancer. The breast cancer itself may not be the cause of the patient's deterioration, but the presence of the cancer makes it such that the body cannot fight the infection. What would the checklist say about this situation?

We can look to Bruce's story as an example. When I first met him as an intern, his disease was close to the point of irreversibility. His infection was so severe there was a good chance he would not have pulled through. He was on life support for a prolonged period of time and endured tremendous suffering. His disease could have taken his life at any point and it certainly would not have been unreasonable to transition his care to comfort measures or hospice care. But his doctors and family pressed on, knowing that infections, even as bad as his, *may* eventually be reversible. Bruce's story demonstrates the element of grey. He had a potentially reversible infection overlaying an irreversible condition (his severe heart failure) since, at the time, Bruce was not a transplant candidate because of his infection, and his heart failure was irreversible in the absence of a transplant. Had Bruce possessed an advance directive saying with a check mark that he did not want mechanical ventilation, would it have applied in this circumstance? It's not so cut and dry as a simple yes/no answer and this demonstrates again how the checkbox advance directive may fail.

After all, end of life decision-making is not about yes/no answers. It's about judgment and scenarios, it's about taking the full picture into consideration and making the best decision possible based on the information we have and what we know about what the patient would want to endure. This is why the advance directive cannot stand as an entity by itself; it cannot exhibit judgment on its own.

Enter the surrogate decision maker.

Surrogate Decision Makers:
Naming Your Go-To Person

Regardless of whether you have an advance directive or not, if you become unable to make your own medical decisions, your medical team should seek out your family for guidance in making decisions for your medical care. Even when an advance directive has been filled out, physicians should not make medical decisions for an incapacitated patient in the absence of consultation with the patients' family. This means, however, that someone will carry the heavy responsibility of speaking for you and helping the doctors to uphold your wishes if you become unable to communicate with your medical team.

Despite the peppering of different terms that exist for this person (health care proxy, power of attorney, surrogate decision maker, next of kin), they all basically mean the same thing: who is going to be the "go-to" person for the medical team? Choosing this person is probably the most important thing you can specify when considering end-of-life planning and is arguably the best way to maintain control and prevent conflict or uncertainty. This decision shouldn't be made lightly, and a lot of different considerations need to go into choosing your decision maker. This person will literally have your life in their hands.

First, however, let's consider what might happen in the absence of an officially named surrogate decision maker. The default go-to person is the legal next of kin, usually the spouse or eldest child, depending on state laws. Most advance directives and living wills have a section in which you can name a power of attorney, who may or may not be the same person as your legal next of kin.

This designation is usually found after the checklist:

I ( )do ( )do not want to designate another person as my surrogate to make medical treatment decisions for me if I should be incompetent and in a terminal condition or in a state of permanent unconsciousness.

Name and address of surrogate (if applicable):

Name and address of substitute surrogate (if surrogate designated above is unable to serve):

I made this declaration on the day of (month, year).

Declarant's signature:

Declarant's address:

The declarant or the person on behalf of and at the direction of the declarant knowingly and voluntarily signed this writing by signature or mark in my presence.

Witness' signature:

Witness' address:

Witness' signature:

Witness' address:

When you name a power of attorney in an advance directive, this designated person's decisions will trump those of the next of kin. So, for example, if you wish to have your best friend make your medical decisions for you rather than your child, you would need to have your friend named as your power of attorney in a legal document.

As long as you've named your "go-to" person in writing, there should not be any doubt about who will be in control of your medical decisions. Theoretically. However, reality and theory often do not coincide. It's equally important to tell your family who the decision maker will be to avoid any surprises when a crisis arises. Surprises are never good in the world of intensive care, and having family members fight and disagree over who will make the final decisions is all too common. Who you've chosen to be your go to person should be clearly communicated to your family, preferably in a time of health. This way, if there is disagreement it can be discussed in a non-emergent setting as opposed to the intensive care unit. Even the most closely knit families may disagree and even though you may hope everyone in your family will come together in a time of crisis, that, unfortunately, is not always the case. Unifying your family behind a single person beforehand will help the doctors take better care of you and also to help your loved ones through a time of crisis when you may not be able to help them otherwise.

Know Your Wishes:
Upholding Your Philosophy

Being someone's medical decision maker is a tough job under any circumstance, particularly when faced with decisions about continuing with aggressive medical care or transitioning care to comfort measures only. It can be agonizing, particularly if your go-to person is not prepared to make the tough choices that will inevitably arise. An unprepared surrogate decision maker is almost as unhelpful as no decision maker at all. Granted, there is no way to predict what situation may arise, but we can make decisions ahead of time about our overall philosophy on end of life care. Just as there are countless variants of religious and moral beliefs in our society, so are there countless variants of how you might feel about the way your body is treated in a time of critical illness and impending death.

In order to appropriately prepare your go-to person for the decisions that lay ahead, you have to know for yourself what you would want under certain general circumstances. After all, how can you possibly expect someone else to figure out what you would want if you don't know for yourself? It's not pleasant to think about our own demise or what might happen if we suddenly became critically ill, but ignoring our own mortality will only make matters even more uncertain. Although it seems daunting, it's important to define your overall philosophy about what kinds of medical care you prefer.

Do this by thinking about what's important to you, and talk about it with your decision maker. Talk about how you feel about independence, about hospitals, about doctors, about awareness, about death, about organ donation.

What matters to you?

What does quality of life mean to you and at what cost are you willing to preserve your bodily functions?

Would you be agreeable to being fed by a tube in order to stay alive?

Would you be agreeable to being unconscious on a ventilator if it meant you were able to keep fighting another day?

How long would you allow your body to be maintained on life support before wanting to succumb or would you want to hold on to life at all costs?

As a unique example, take Patrick, the teenager who, after a lifetime of being a slave to cystic fibrosis, was able to gain control and peace in his final months. Those who knew Patrick knew that his decision to stop aggressive treatment and enroll in hospice care, even at the age of nineteen, was in line with the way that he desired his life to be: independent of nebulizers, cystic fibrosis medications and machines. Once he was diagnosed with the dreaded superbug, cepacia, he reached a turning point in his life in which he was able to regain control and live out the rest of his life on his own terms, based on his definition of quality of life. His personal philosophy wouldn't tolerate his final months being spent among doctors, hidden away in hospitals and isolation rooms. To his family and friends who had observed Patrick's lifelong struggle for normality, his choice seemed obvious. Because Patrick was able to successfully define his philosophy of quality of life and to set clear boundaries for his medical care, his final months were spent exactly as he envisioned.

With medical decision-making, there's no absolute right or wrong answer, only what is right or wrong for you. Taking *most* of the guess work out of the equation can be achieved, but only if you talk to your decision maker, loved ones and doctors about your general philosophy. Your discussion will build the foundation they will need to make your decisions. Without it, your decision makers will be left without your voice to make tough choices, which, without the appropriate level of preparedness, may be even more difficult and painful than the grief of losing a loved one.

Engage With Grace

Alexandra Drane and Matthew Holt created the movement Engage With Grace (www.engagewithgrace.org) with the mission of empowering others to start talking about the issues we all tend avoid. Engage With Grace brings to focus these fundamental issues by encouraging all of us to address just five basic questions to help better understand, communicate and have our end of life preferences honored. After reading *LAST WISH*, perhaps you are closer to finding the answers that will help you to Engage With Grace by answering these five simple, yet actionable questions:

Can You and Your Loved Ones Answer These Questions?

1. On a scale of 1 to 5, where do you fall on this continuum?

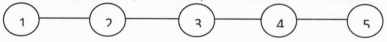

1   2   3   4   5

Let me die without medical intervention

Don't give up on me no matter what, try any proven and unproven intervention possible

2. If there were a choice, would you prefer to die at home, or in a hospital?

3. Could a loved one correctly describe how you'd like to be treated in the case of a terminal illness?

4. Is there someone you trust whom you've appointed to advocate on your behalf when the time is near?

5. Have you completed any of the following: written a living will, appointed a healthcare power of attorney, or completed an advance directive?

ENGAGE WITH GRACE   **engagewithgrace.org**

The One Slide Project

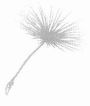

Last Wish Compass:
A Discussion Guide

The task I've set before you is by no means a simple one. Conversations with your loved ones and decision makers about death and dying don't come easily. The five questions of Engage With Grace are simple by design, but they involve a deep and complex emotional understanding of what quality of life may mean for each of us. The conversation that needs to occur between a person and his or her chosen decision maker is intimate and may be uncomfortable to initiate and even intimidating. It takes more than the intention to have the conversation; it takes courage and a little bit of guidance. Although it's ideal to have end-of-life conversations with your physicians and health care professionals, you may want to start thinking about these issues before arriving at your physician's office, and the tools in this book are designed to help you do just that.

To help you accomplish this, I've created the Last Wish Compass, a discussion guide meant to aid you and your surrogates as you navigate the five questions of Engage With Grace and other end-of-life choices you should consider. The Compass is meant to stimulate discussion between you and your family, not to replace the creation of formal advance directives or the naming of a power of attorney. Use it together as a way to determine limits to life-sustaining treatments and to help you answer the question: what is a meaningful quality of life for me? Tear it out of the book, write on it, show it to your loved ones and your physicians, and use it as a talking piece about the scenarios on the Compass. Start preparing yourself and your loved ones now, before it's too late.

Discussion Questions for
The Last Wish Compass

1. Why is it so difficult for patients, families and clinicians to initiate end-of-life discussions?

2. How is the Last Wish Compass (pages 171-173) different than a typical advance directive (page 162). What does the Compass cover that goes beyond information in an advance directive?

3. Why might the Last Wish Compass be a useful addition to an advance directive or living will?

The Last Wish Compass: A Discussion Guide

This document is meant to serve as a guide for my family if they are faced with making decisions for me if and when I become unable to do so myself. It is meant to supplement, not replace, the legal documentation of Advance Directives and to help clarify my personal interpretation of the phrase "meaningful quality of life," which varies from person to person.

1. **Place a check in the box next to the approximate time you consider to be "too long" on full life support (ie. a breathing machine or ventilator) which would require you to be in a coma-like state (ie. sedated and/or unable to interact with others.**

   ☐ No amount of time. I do not want life support.   ☐ Days   ☐ Weeks   ☐ Months   ☐ Indefinitely

2. **Imagine that you are seriously ill with a condition that is ultimately terminal with a small chance of recovery and little to no hope of a cure. Place a check mark in the box that most accurately reflects your level of agreement with each statement on the left.**

	Unacceptable. This is not what I consider an acceptable quality of life.	This is an acceptable but not desirable quality of life. I could accept this condition for: Days · Weeks · Months			Fully acceptable. I could still have a high quality of life in this condition.
I am not able to return to my home.					
I am unable to chew or swallow food or liquid. I require artificial nutrition through a feeding tube.					
I am awake but unable to communicate or interact with those around me.					
I am not able to walk.					
I am dependent on others to help me perform simple daily activities (going to bathroom, getting out of bed and into a chair).					

continued on next page

For more info on Last Wish Compass, visit www.knowyourwishes.com

Last Wish Compass: A Discussion Guide, page 2

2. (*continued*)

	Unacceptable. This is not what I consider an acceptable quality of life.	This is an acceptable but not desirable quality of life. I could accept this condition for: Days Weeks Months			Fully acceptable. I could still have a high quality of life in this condition.
I require a semi-permanent or permanent tracheostomy (ie. surgical tube in my neck) to stay connected to the breathing machine but I am awake, alert and pain free.					
I am not able to remember or recognize my family.					
I am being kept alive as long as modern medicine allows, even though I am unaware of my surroundings, in significant pain, and with little to no hope of recovery.					

3. Place a check in the box next to the phrase that best describes your feelings about cardiopulmonary resuscitation (CPR), a process where doctors use shocks or manually compress the heart to restart it if it stops beating. I understand that this would require me to be placed at least temporarily on a breathing machine.

☐ I would want CPR even if there was only a minimal chance I might regain a meaningful quality of life, but it kept me alive.

☐ I would want CPR if there was a decent chance I might recover to a meaningful quality of life.

☐ I would decline CPR, and prefer to allow natural death.

4. I have completed a separate Power of Attorney and have named the following person to make my medical decisions if I am unable.

Name   Relationship   Date

This is not a legal document.

For more info on Last Wish Compass, visit www.knowyourwishes.com

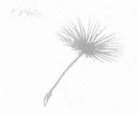

Discussion Questions

Last Wish:
Stories to Inspire a Peaceful Passing

1. What inspired you to read Last Wish?

2. Do you have any personal stories or experiences with critical illness or end-of-life care? How did this experience affect you?

3. Have you ever considered the way you would want your medical care handled if you were seriously ill? Why or why not?

The Last Wish Compass

1. Why is it so difficult for patients, families and clinicians to initiate end-of-life discussions?

2. How is the Last Wish Compass (pages 184-185) different than a typical advance directive (page 171). What does the Compass cover that goes beyond information in an advance directive?

3. Why might the Last Wish Compass be a useful addition to an advance directive or living will?

A Biker's Heart

1. Bruce was in a state of near death for many months and endured many invasive procedures prior to getting his heart transplant. What were the trade-offs for Bruce and his family as they continued full aggressive medical therapy? What sacrifices did he make in order to survive his illness?

2. Bruce was a middle aged, strong and healthy man prior to his life threatening illness. Consider how a person's condition prior to serious illness influences their ability to recover. How should this impact decisions made about invasive and aggressive medical interventions?

3. What would you be willing to give up in order to survive a life-threatening illness (discomfort, independence, ability to eat, walk, etc)? What would you not be willing to sacrifice?

Breathless

1. How did you feel and what emotions did you experience when reading Mrs. Chandler's story?

2. Much of Mrs. Chandler's story could have been different if she and her family were more prepared for the terminal nature of her illness. Why do you suppose there was so much conflict and turmoil surrounding her end-of-life experience? Consider the role of a living will or advanced directive?

3. Lisa and Sam had difficulty recognizing that Mrs. Chandler would not recover from her terminal cancer. What role does hope serve for families facing terminal illness or the impending loss of a loved one?

4. Lisa and Sam's religious faith influenced the medical decisions they made for their mother. Consider and discuss the role of faith in medicine and science.

5.   Lisa said that Mrs. Chandler wanted "to live." Think about what "living" and quality of life mean to you. How would you want to be cared for if you were in Mrs. Chandler's situation? What would you want your family to know?

A Courageous Choice

1.   Patrick knew where his "line in the sand" was and courageously faced it—where is your line in the sand? Why is it important to communicate your wishes to your family and how might you go about doing so?

2.   Were you surprised to hear Patrick ask his physician about hospice? What was your initial reaction about Patrick enrolling on hospice? Was his experience what you expected? Would you feel comfortable discussing hospice with your physician if you had a terminal disease? Why or why not?

3.   Although Patrick was young, his story shows us the reality of people living with chronic, yet ultimately terminal illnesses. What did you learn from Patrick's experience?

The Heart of the Matter

1.   Why do you think it was hard for Walter's parents to understand to that he was dead, but still had vital signs on the monitor?

2.   Once the doctors declared Walter brain dead, his parents had no end-of-life decisions to make, even though his heart was still beating. Why is this situation so unique?

3.   How did you conceptualize the moment of death prior to reading Walter's story? How did his story change your perception, if at all?

The Hospice Bride

1. After reading Barbara's story, did your perceptions of hospice care and its benefits change and if so, how?

2. There are many misconceptions about hospice care. Think about and discuss how Barbara's experience is contrary to the following misconceptions:

    a. Hospice care means stopping all medical therapies and medications.
    b. Being on hospice means you're giving up.
    c. People who enroll on hospice always die within a short period of time.
    d. Hospice is very expensive.

3. Some say hospice is a way to die, but Barbara says that it is instead a way to live. How do you feel about the idea of hospice care?

A Peaceful Passing

1. Victoria's family was faced with an unexpected decision in a crisis situation. What would you have done if you were her daughters?

2. Ultimately, Victoria's family was guided by her values and preferences when it came to medical decision-making—what would you want your family to consider?

3. Modern medicine can keep the human body functioning in the setting of very serious illness, however just because we can intervene, does it mean we always should? What are the costs to patients, their families and the healthcare system?

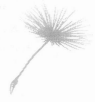

Where to Go for
More Information

Last Wish is by no means a comprehensive guide to end-of-life care and planning. I encourage you to use this book and its tools to begin thinking about the scenarios and establish your own principles, and to spend some time reflecting on the way these stories made you feel and the opinions you formed as you read the experiences of these five patients. Talk to your loved ones and family about your reflections, and try to open a discussion about these topics we tend to avoid. Prepare yourself, prepare your family, and prepare your doctors with the tools they'll need to carry through your wishes and your legacy.

Visit www.knowyourwishes.com for discussion boards, information and resources about Last Wish and medical decision-making.

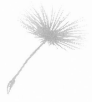

Acknowledgments

Last Wish could not have been written without the help, support, and encouragement of my mentors, family, and friends. From the conception of this project to the implementation, I have been blessed with a strong network surrounding me that has enabled this book to take shape.

Last Wish would not exist if it weren't for Dr. Jill Bolte Taylor, whose response to a simple email made a project that seemed like a pipe dream become a possibility. I am incredibly thankful for the work of Ellen Stiefler of Transmedia Books for taking me under her wing, believing in this project, and guiding me through the world of publishing. I am also deeply appreciative for the editing talent of Karen Risch.

I give thanks to the mentorship of Dr. Michael Sherman not only for his guidance throughout this project and my career thus far, but also through life. I am especially grateful for the mentorship and friendship of Dr. Richard Paluzzi, who I can always count on for his honesty, integrity and perspective. I am also fortunate for the mentorship and encouragement of Dr. Robert Promisloff, as well as countless other faculty, nurses, case managers, and friends I've made at Drexel University College of Medicine and Hahnemann University Hospital.

Thanks go to the physicians, patients, nurses and family members who granted me interviews to ensure the accuracy of this work as well as to help me capture the color of the people who make up the stories of Last Wish and to Alicia Bloom for helping me focus my message.

I'd also like to thank my entire family, from my husband, Mike, to my amazingly supportive parents, Michael Pitkow and Barbara Healy, as well as my wonderful stepparents, Tim Healy and Jane Schreiber. Thanks go to my brothers Xaq and Sam Pitkow and all of my very special in-laws. An extra thank you goes to my dad and Pitkow Associates for work on design, website, marketing and overall encouragement along with my brother Xaq for his design expertise.

Lastly, I'd like to thank my patients and their families, past, present and future for the honor of treating them through their struggles and victories.

Made in the USA
Charleston, SC
20 December 2012